This is Breck

Written by Mark Harrington

Illustrated by Sydney Johnson

Salamander Street

First published in 2021 by Salamander Street Ltd.
(info@salamanderstreet.com)

ISBN: 9781913630683

Printed and bound in Great Britain

10 9 8 7 6 5 4 3 2 1

Contents

About the Breck Foundation

The Breck Foundation is a charity founded by Lorin LaFave, whose 14-year-old son, Breck, was groomed online and murdered in 2014.

Breck and his friends were groomed by an 18 year old who ran an internet gaming server. They were told an elaborate web of lies to gain their trust. Despite many attempts to stop her son from contacting the predator, and to alert him to the fact that he was being groomed, Lorin was unable to prevent her son's murder.

As a result of the tragedy, Lorin founded the Breck Foundation, determined that no other family should have to go through the same ordeal. The charity now delivers powerful presentations using Breck's story as an example; our impact statement has these numbers: more than 16,000 students, 2,000 parents and 4,000 safeguarding professionals - please change to reflect.

Lorin believes that had her son seen the kind of talk that the Foundation now presents to schools, he would still be alive today.

The Foundation wants to ensure that no child is harmed through grooming and exploitation while enjoying their time on the internet. Prevention through education is essential.

The charity's 'play virtual, live real' motto reminds everyone to never meet up alone in a private place with someone they have met only online.

For further information and resources, please visit **www.breckfoundation.org**

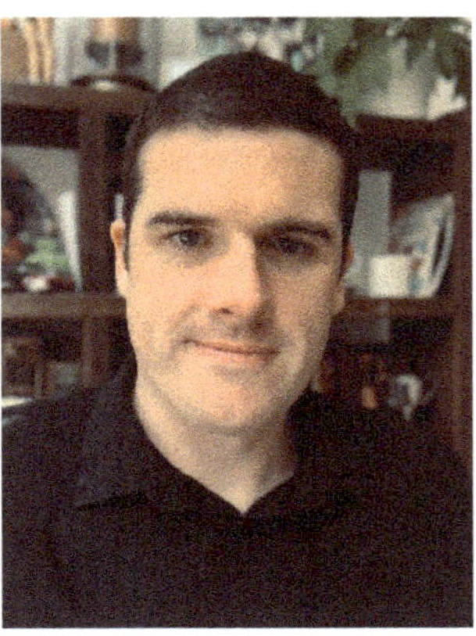

About the Author, Mark Harrington

Mark Harrington is a special needs teacher with more than 10 years' experience in SEN education. He specialises in drama and English adaptions for special needs education. Mark is a trustee for the Breck Foundation, developing educational resources for the charity. For more of Mark's projects please see Instagram @harrington_projects

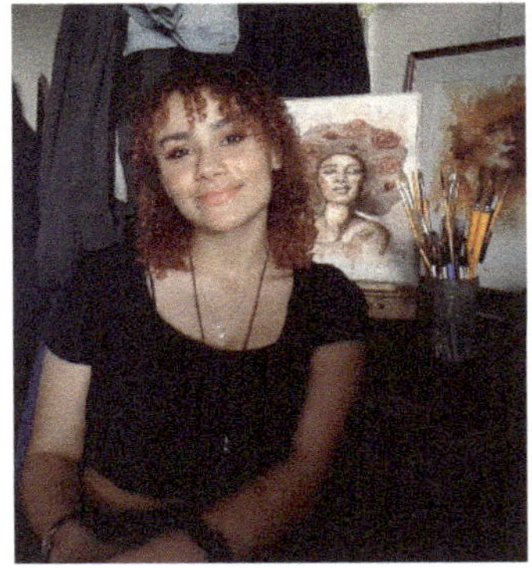

About the Illustrator, Sydney Johnson

Sydney studied art and design at Brighton MET and gained a foundation diploma focusing on illustration. She is a traditional artist working mainly in watercolour, and loves making colourful and expressive portraits of people and animals. Sydney is extremely proud and honoured to be a part of this project and to help spread the word about Breck's story.

Instagram: @syd.c.j

Facebook: Sydney-Johnson-Art

Etsy: SydneyJohnsonArt

For

The students of Manor Green College

&

In memory of Breck Bednar

This is Breck.

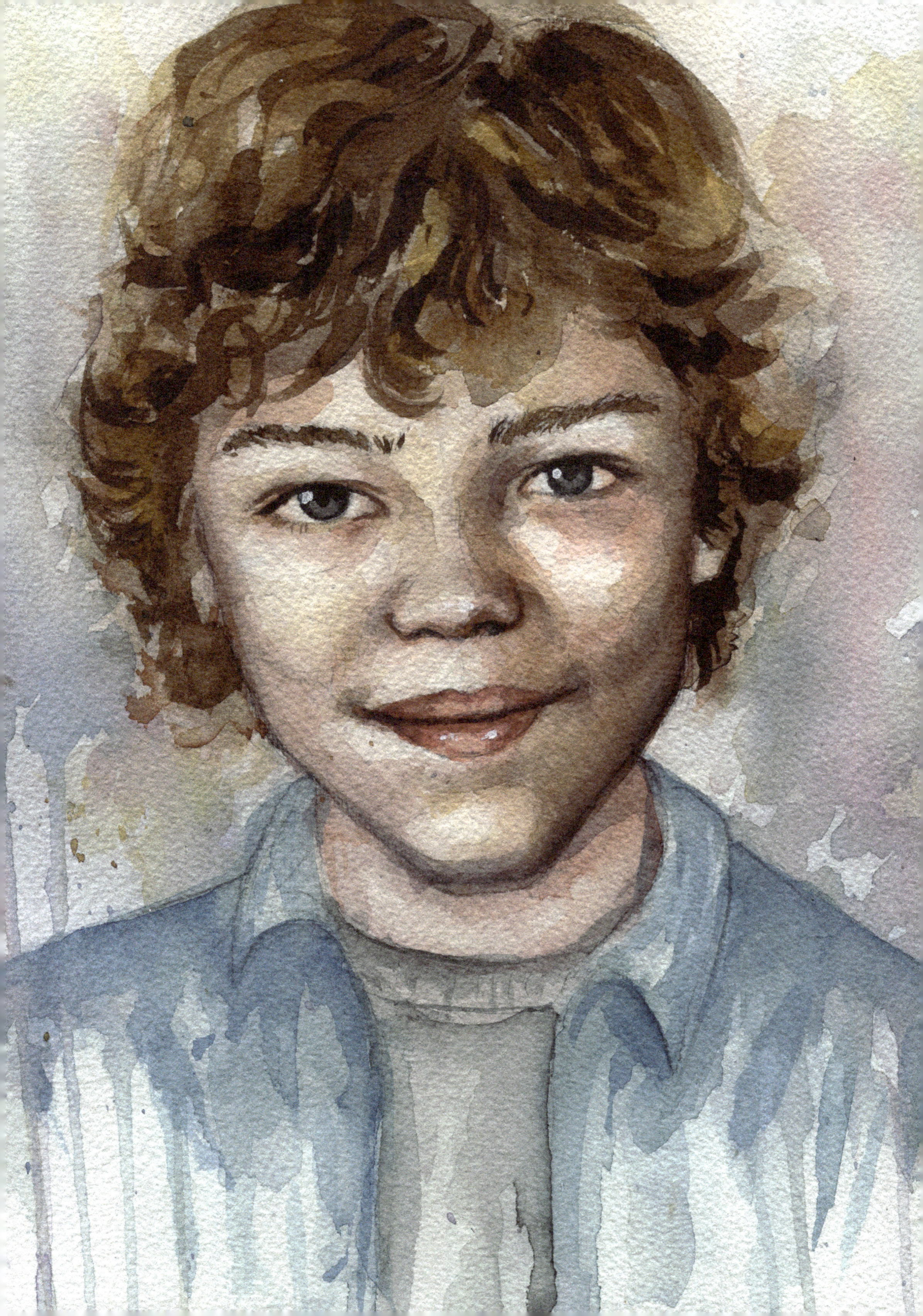

Breck liked to play on the computer.

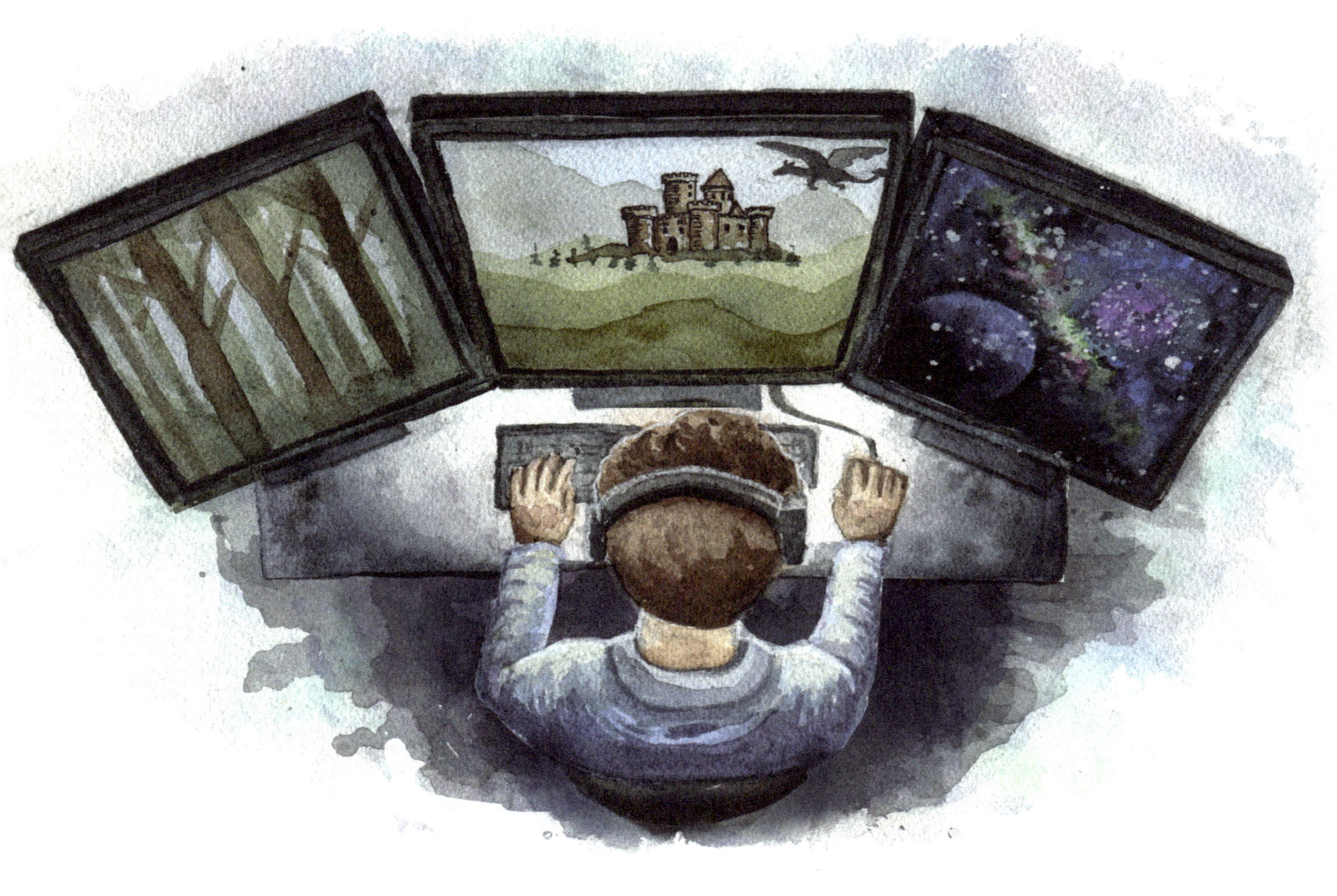

Breck played with his friends on the computer.

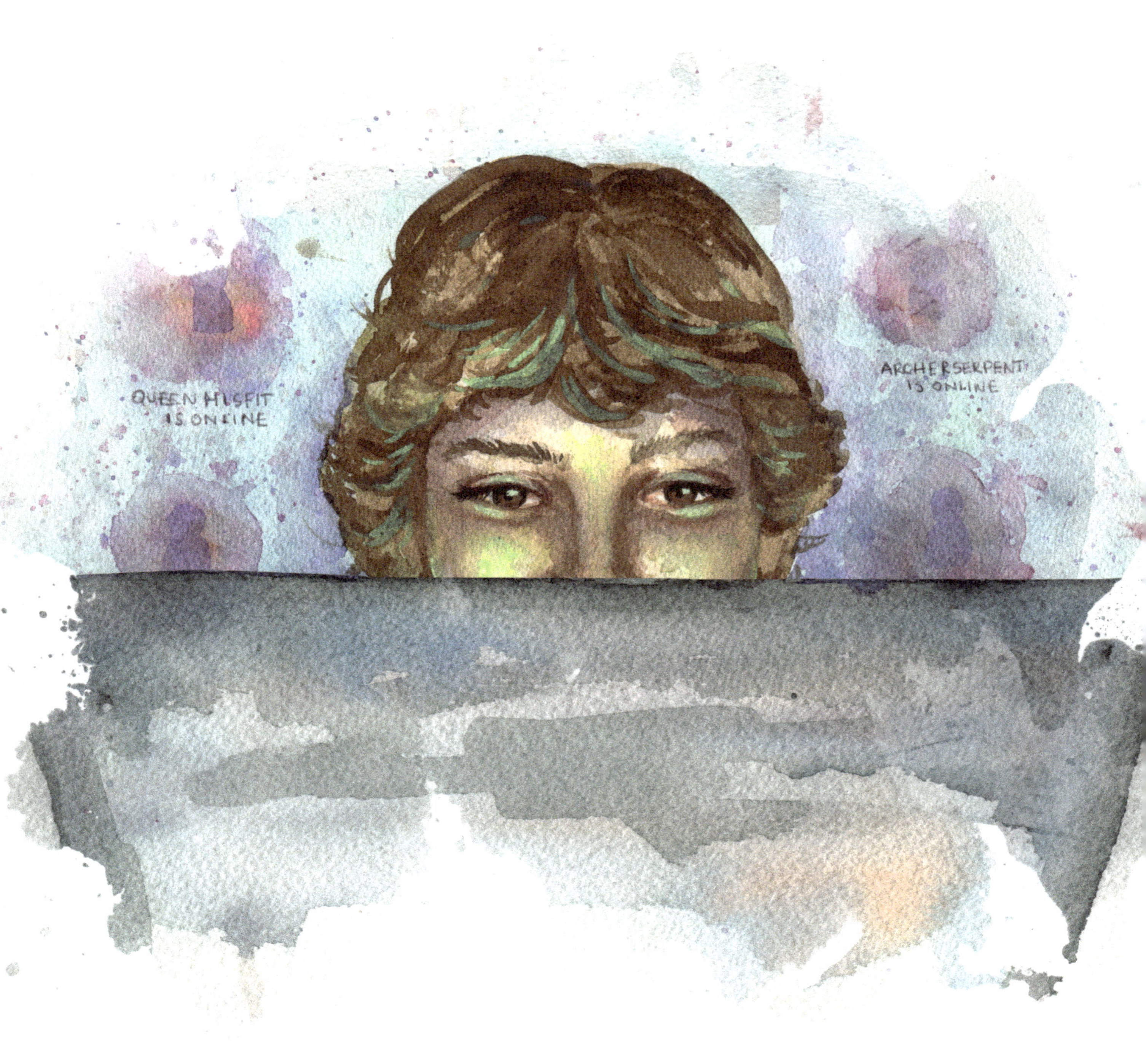

QUEEN MISFIT
IS ONLINE
ARCHERSERPENT
IS ONLINE

Breck made a friend online on the computer but he did not know him.

This person was Lewis.

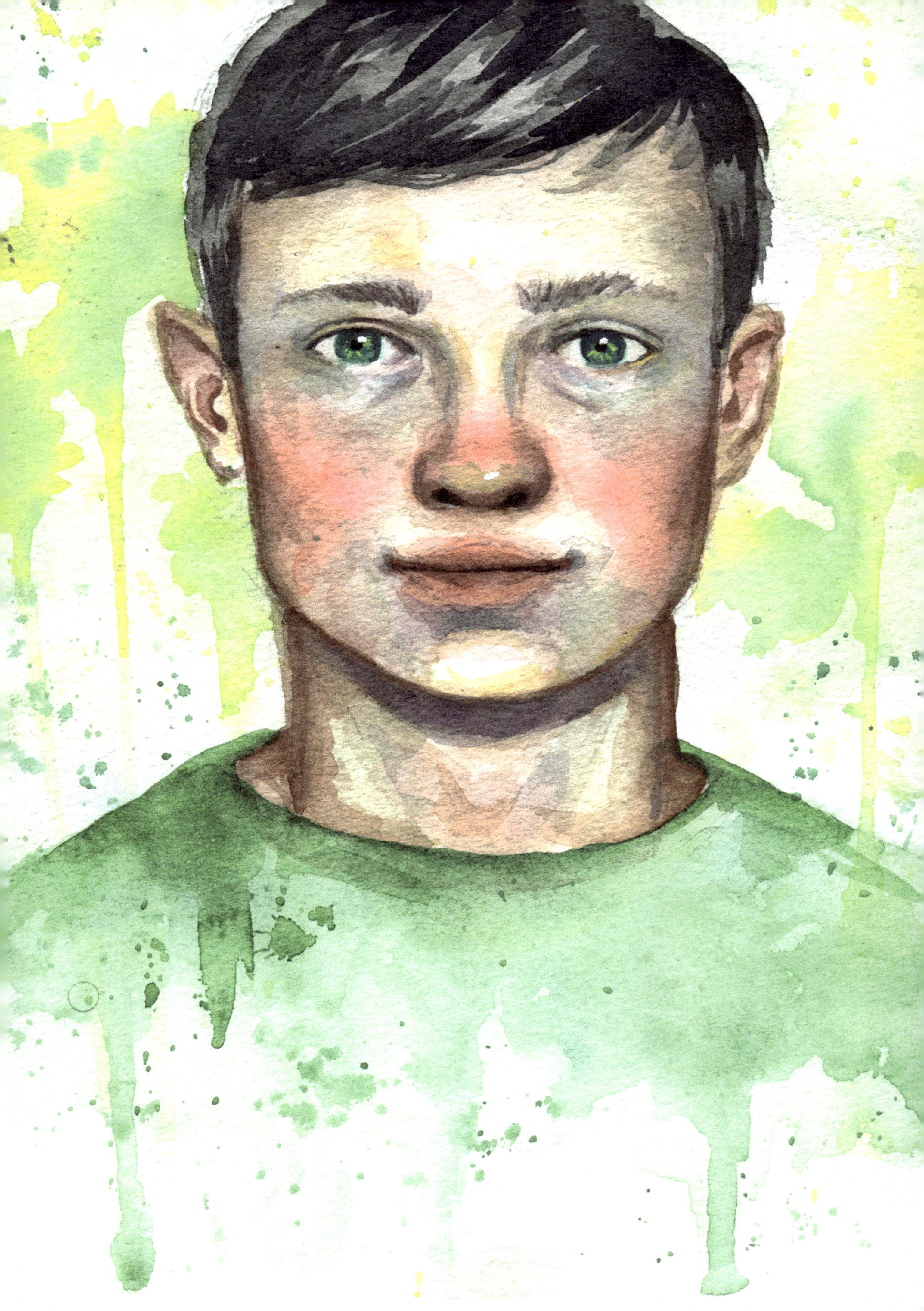

Breck never met Lewis.

They only spoke online or on the computer.

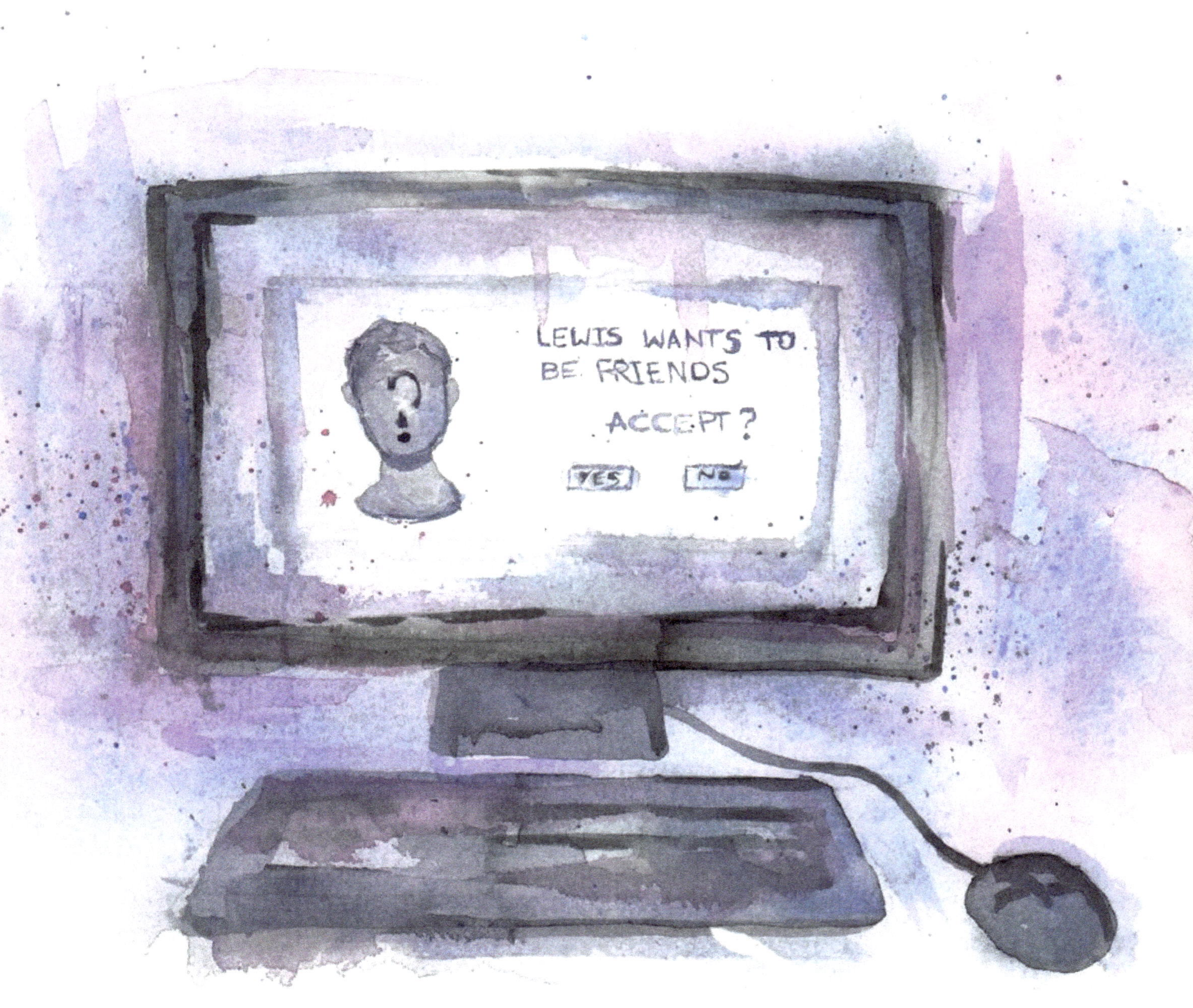

LEWIS WANTS TO BE FRIENDS
ACCEPT ?
YES
NO

Lewis told lies like: he had lots of money,
he had a good job, and he lived in a big house.

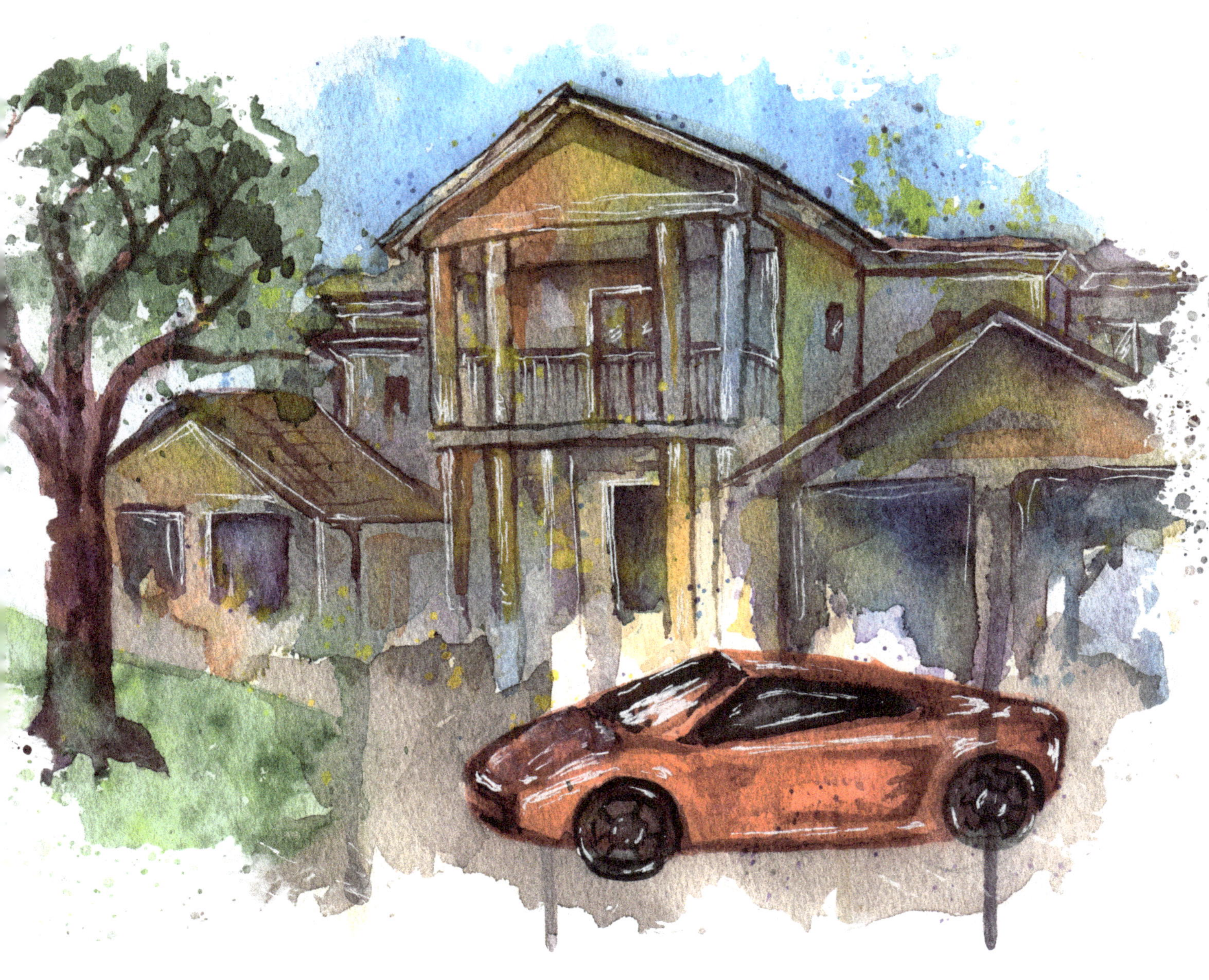

Breck liked Lewis.

Lewis made Breck feel good.

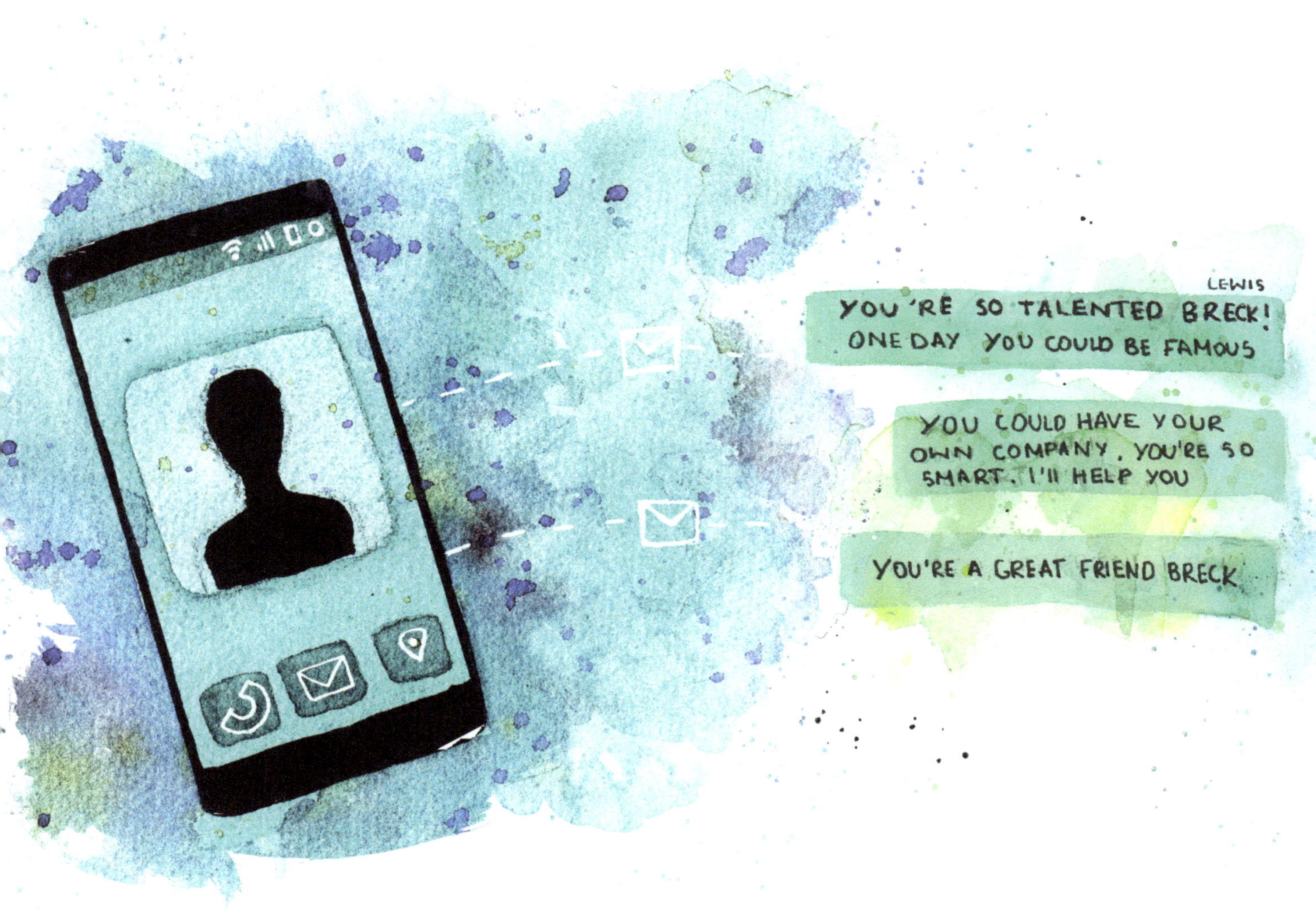

LEWIS
YOU'RE SO TALENTED BRECK! ONE DAY YOU COULD BE FAMOUS
YOU COULD HAVE YOUR OWN COMPANY. YOU'RE SO SMART. I'll HELP YOU
YOU'RE A GREAT FRIEND BRECK

Breck's Mum did not like Breck
and Lewis's friendship.

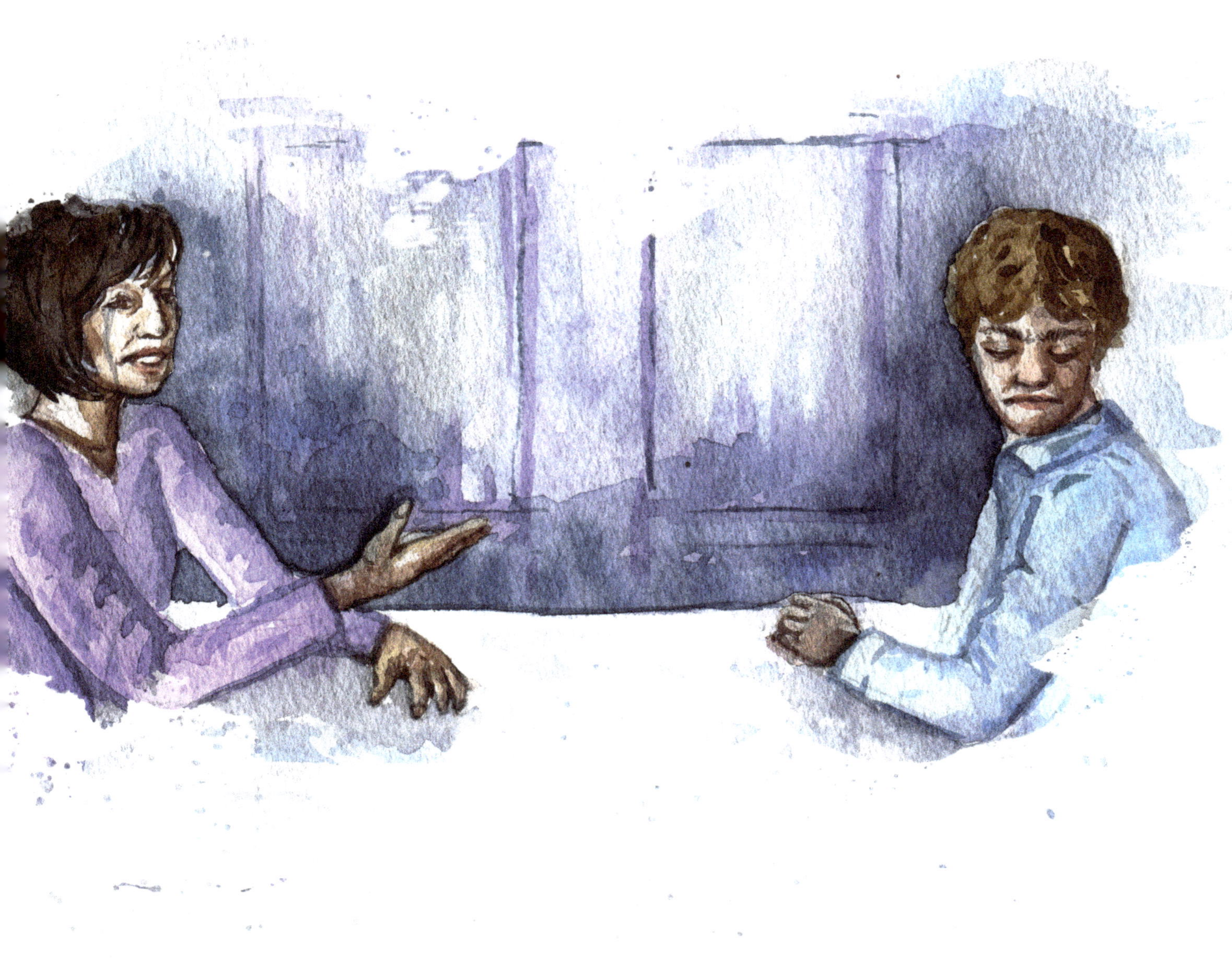

**Breck's other friends did not like
Breck and Lewis's friendship.**

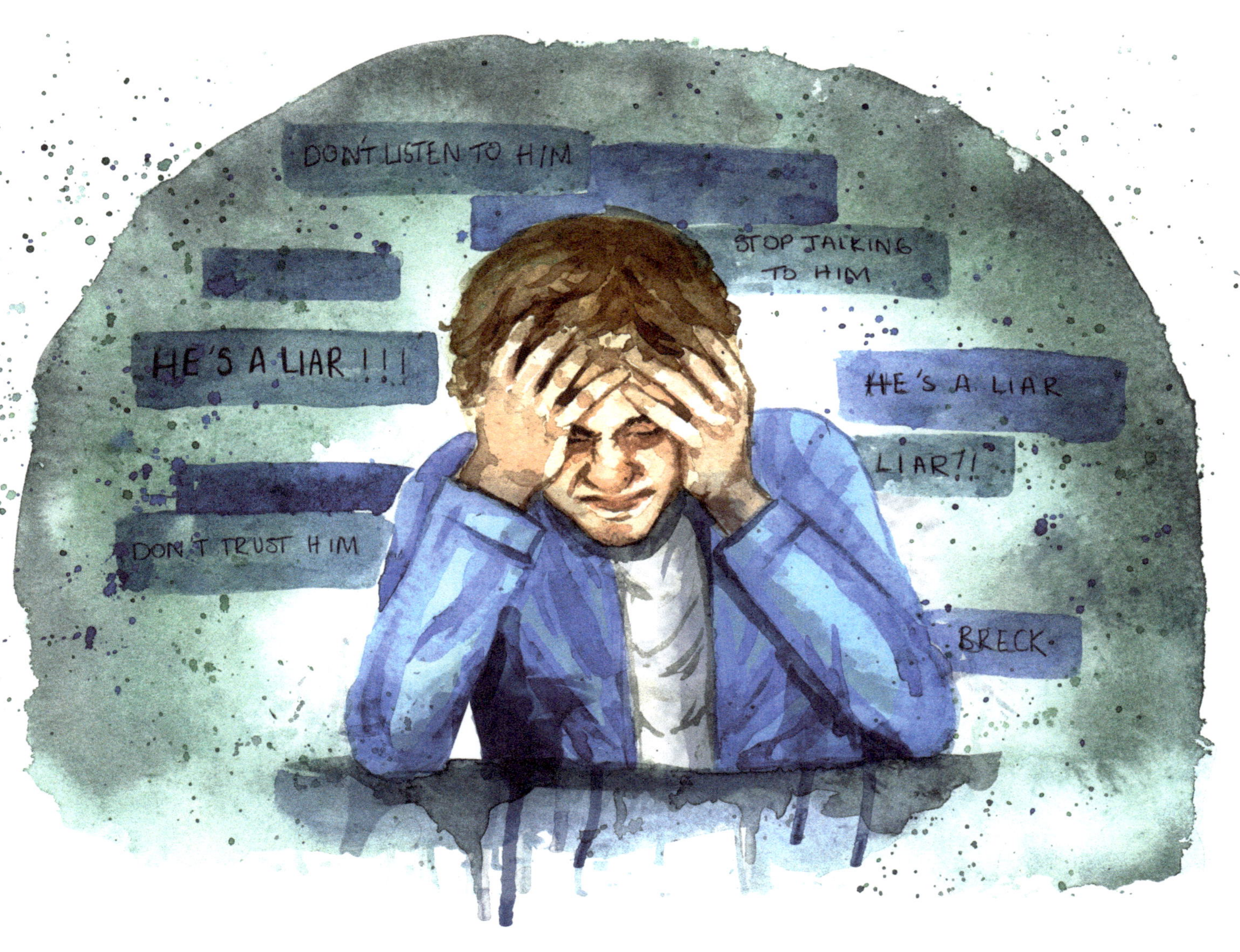

DON'T LISTEN TO HIM
STOP TALKING TO HIM
HE'S A LIAR !!!
HE'S A LIAR
LIAR?!
DON'T TRUST HIM
BRECK

Lewis invited Breck to his house.

Lewis told Breck not to tell his Mum.

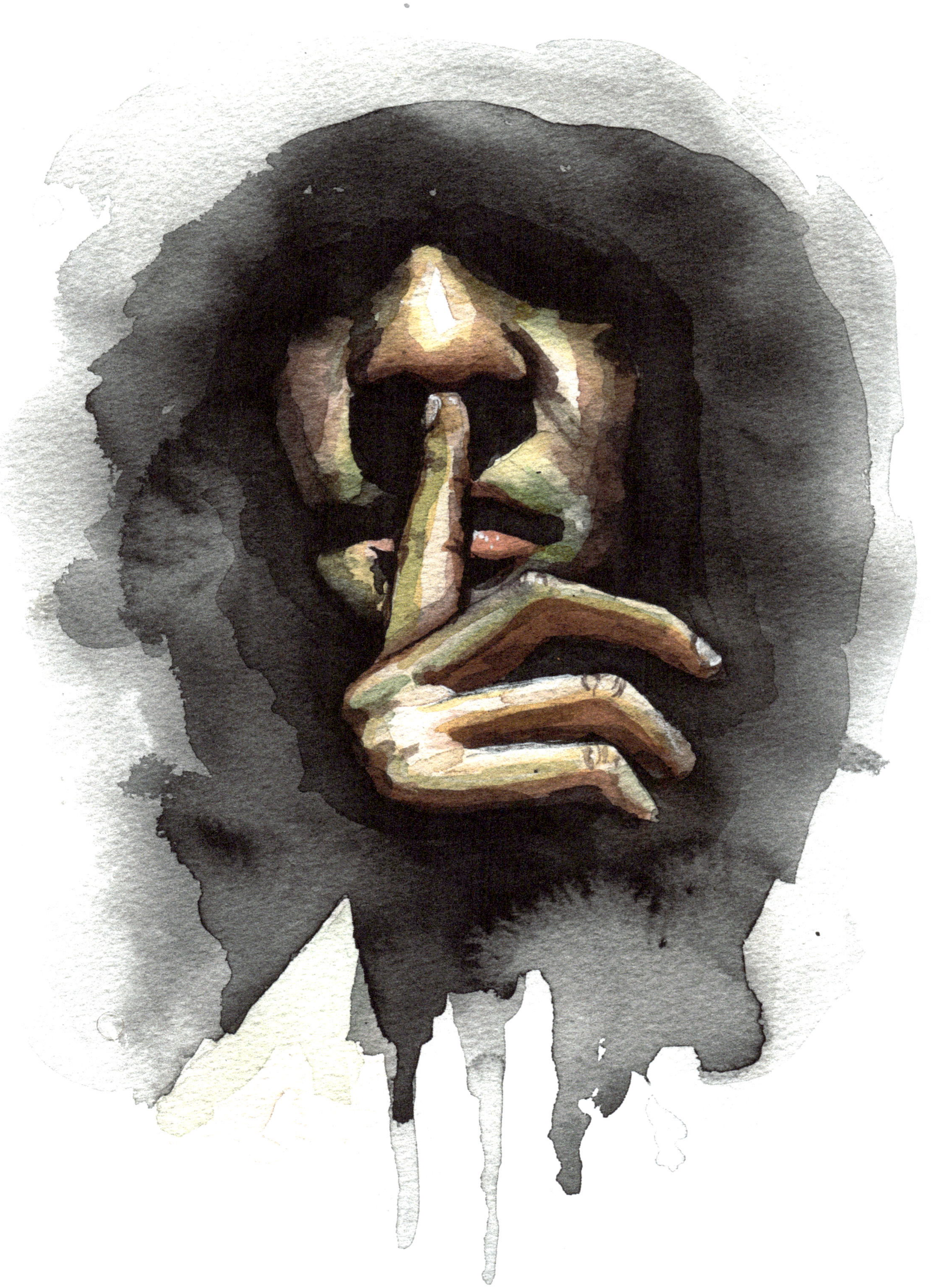

**Breck went to Lewis's house
and did not tell his Mum he was going.**

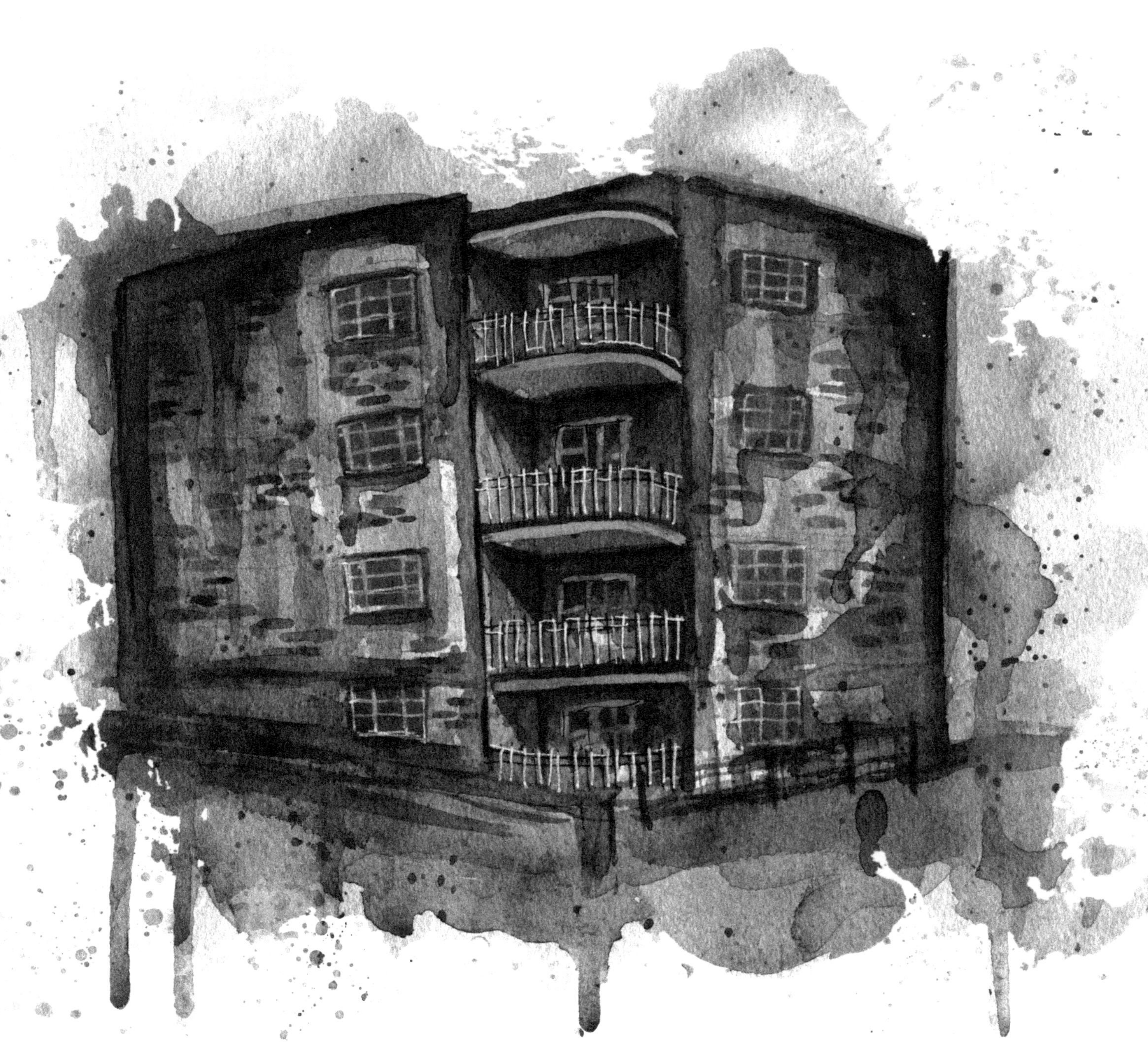

Breck never came out.

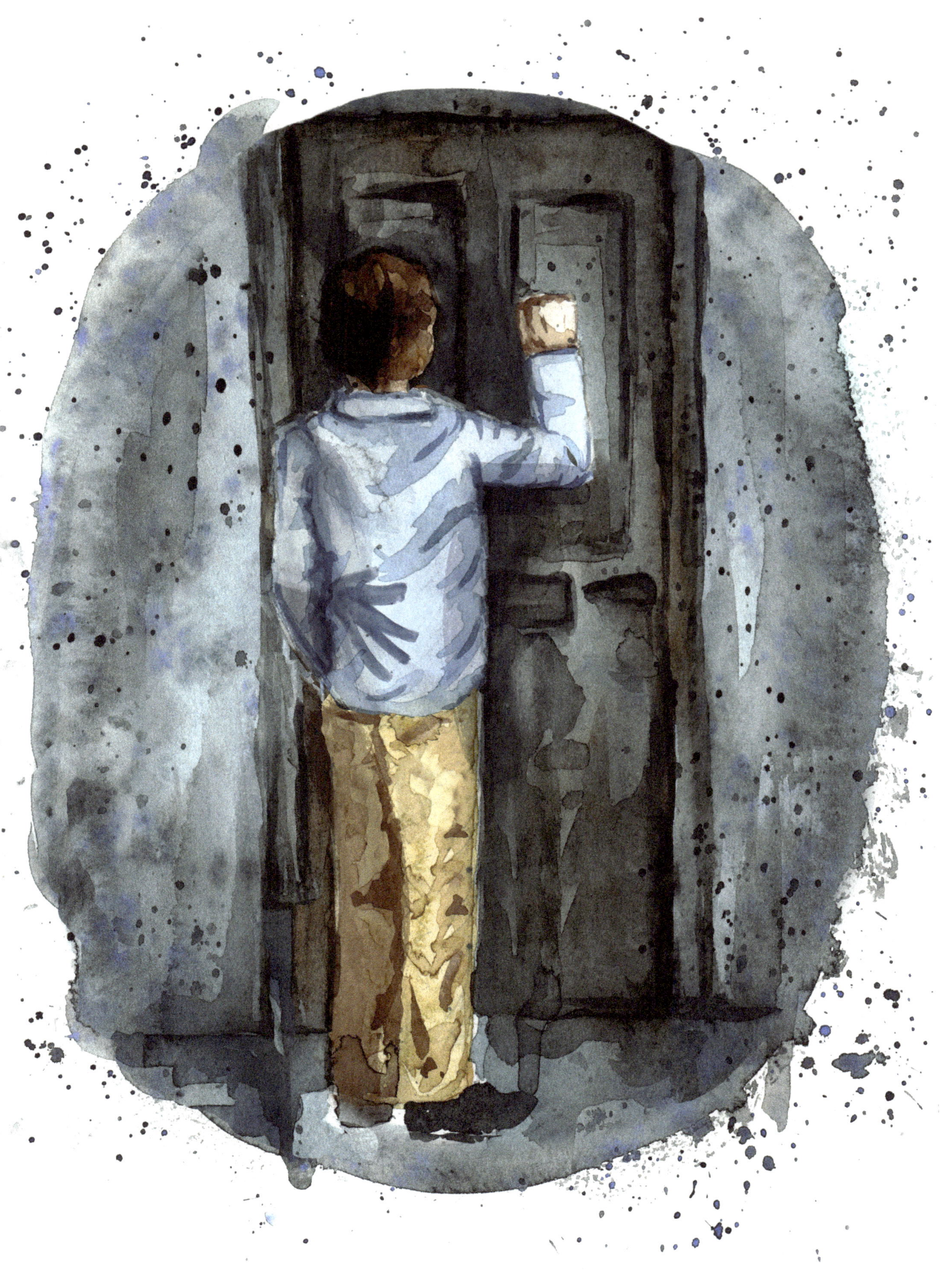

Lewis killed Breck.

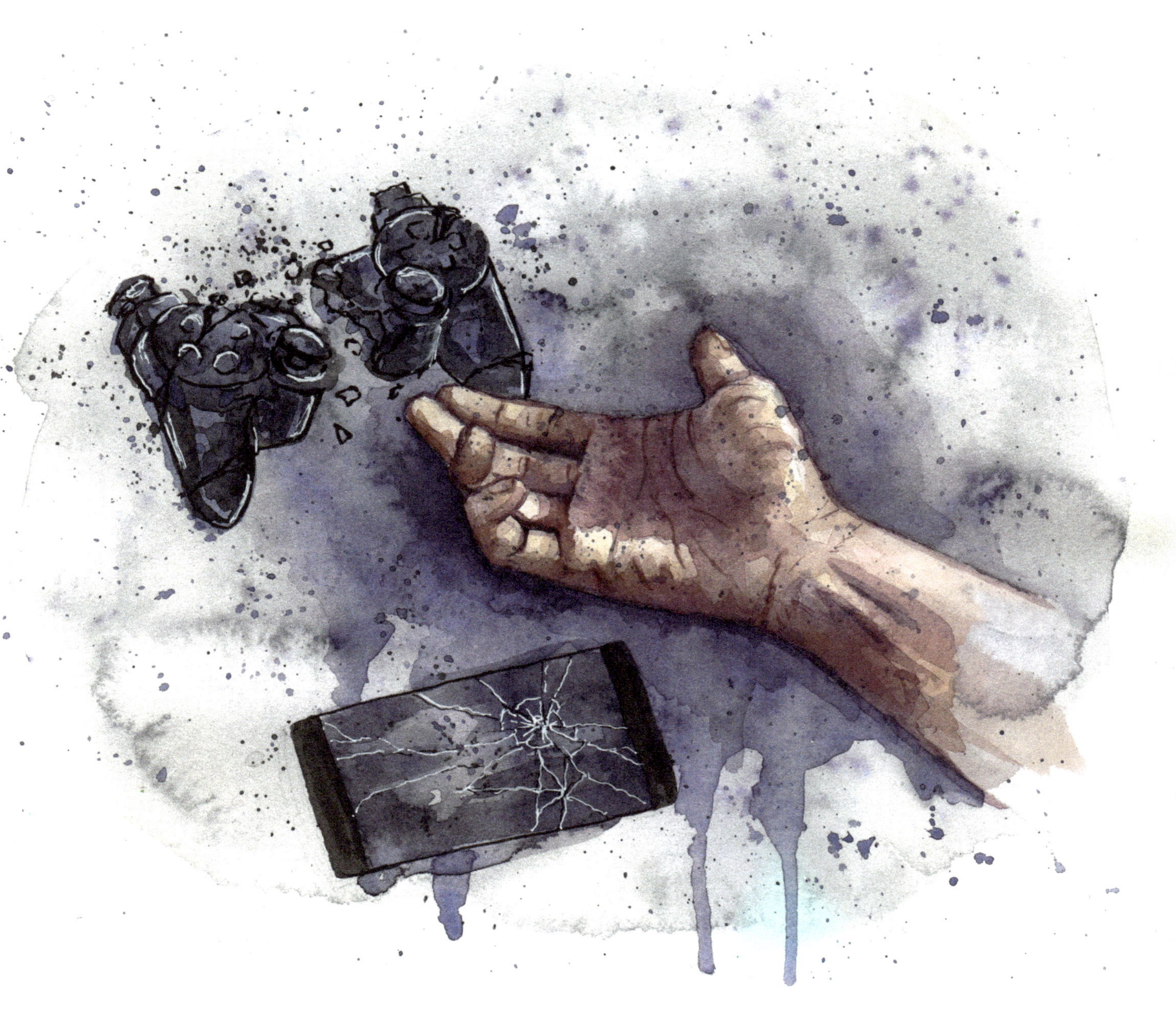

Lewis told lies. Lewis did not have lots of money, he did not have a good job and he did not live in a big house.

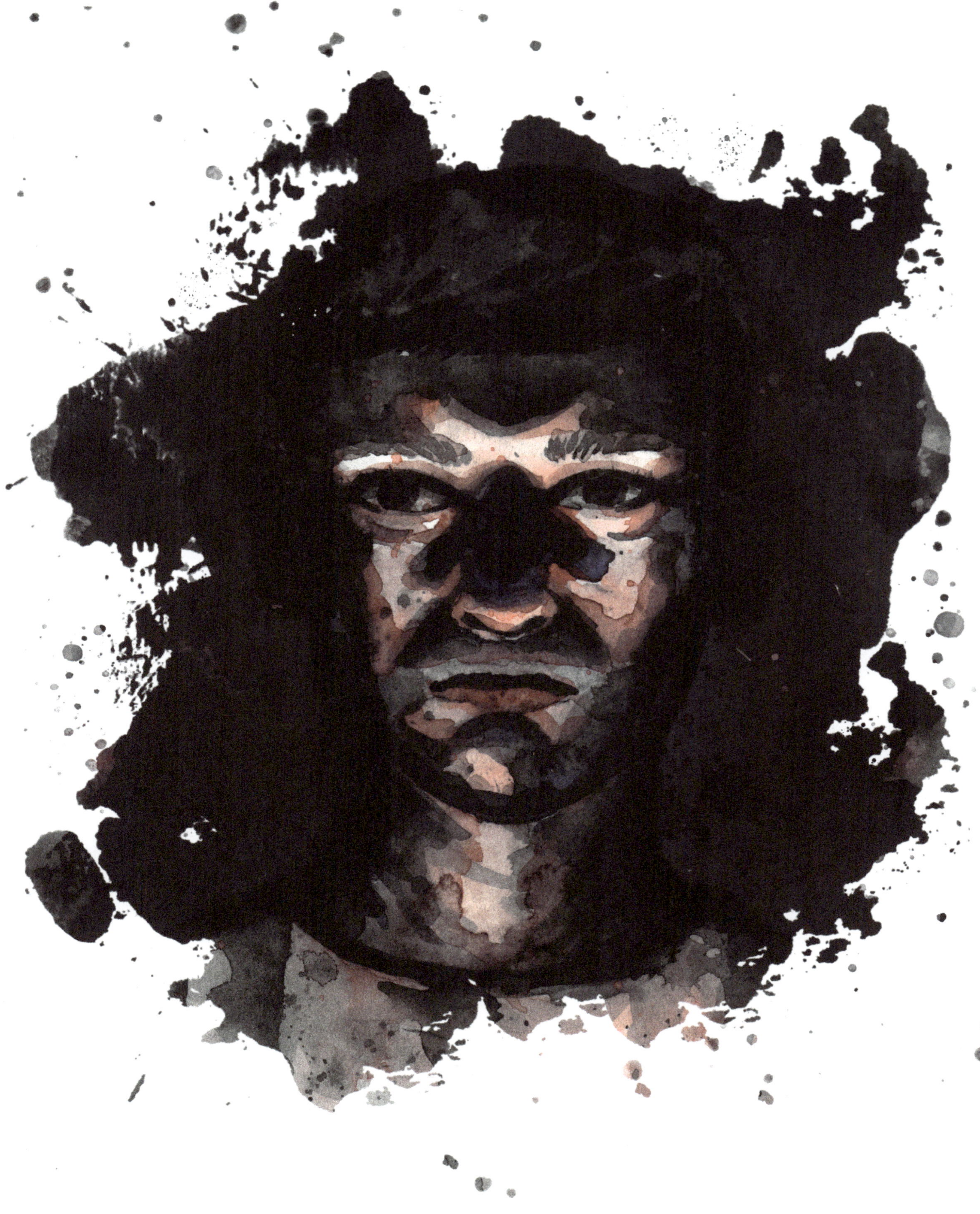

Lewis has gone to prison.

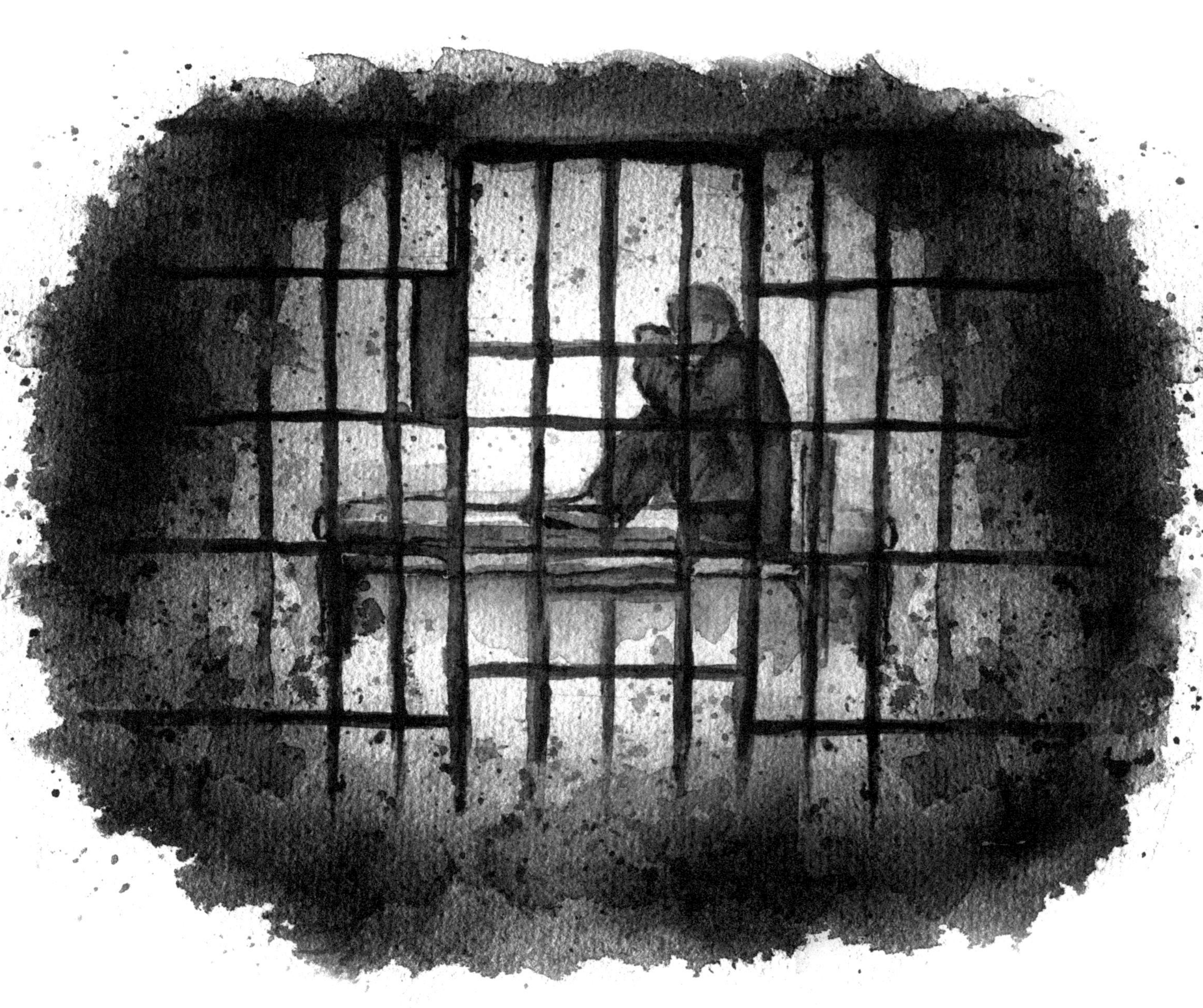

Breck's family are sad and miss Breck.

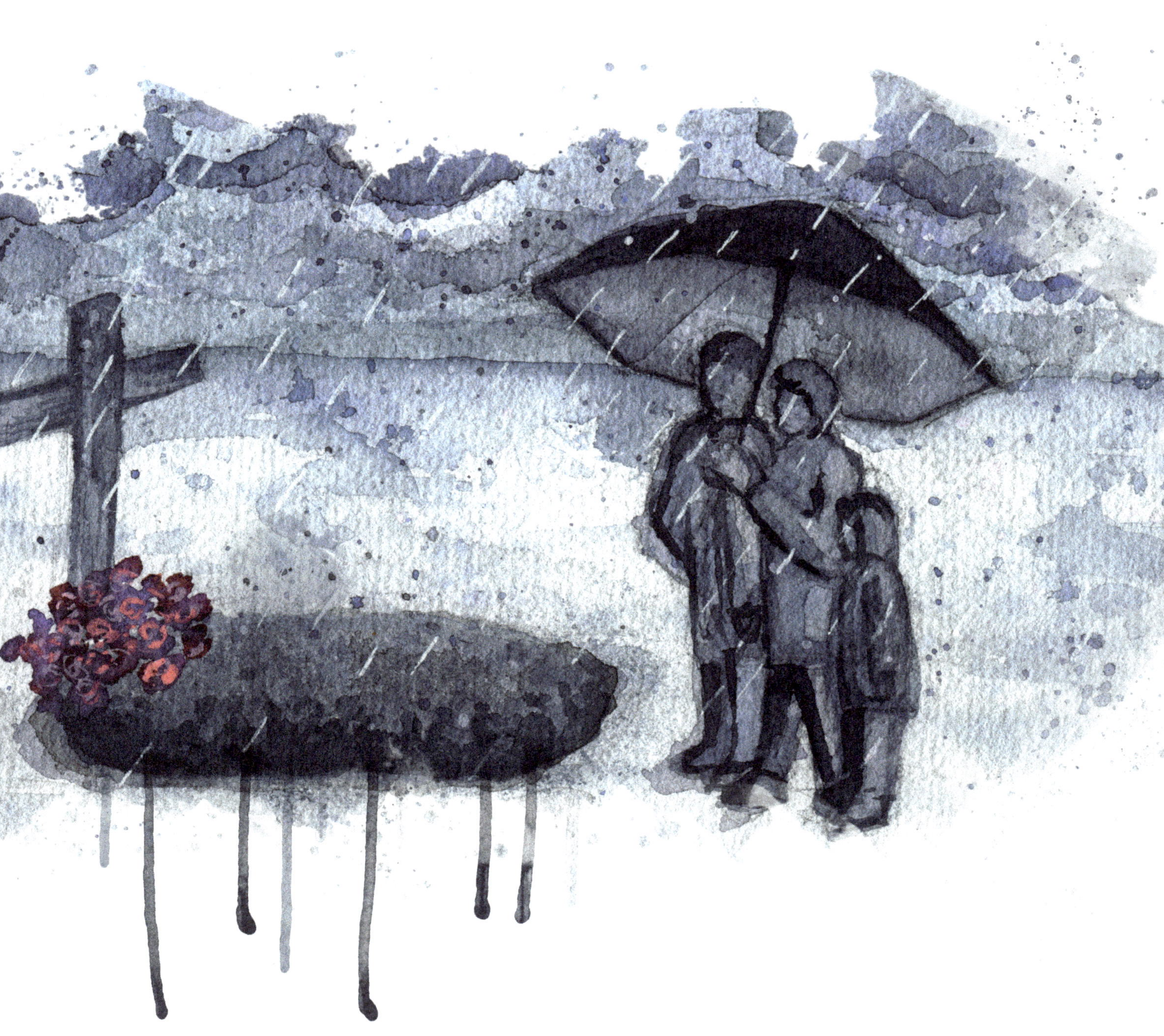

Breck should not have made friends online on the computer with people he did not know.

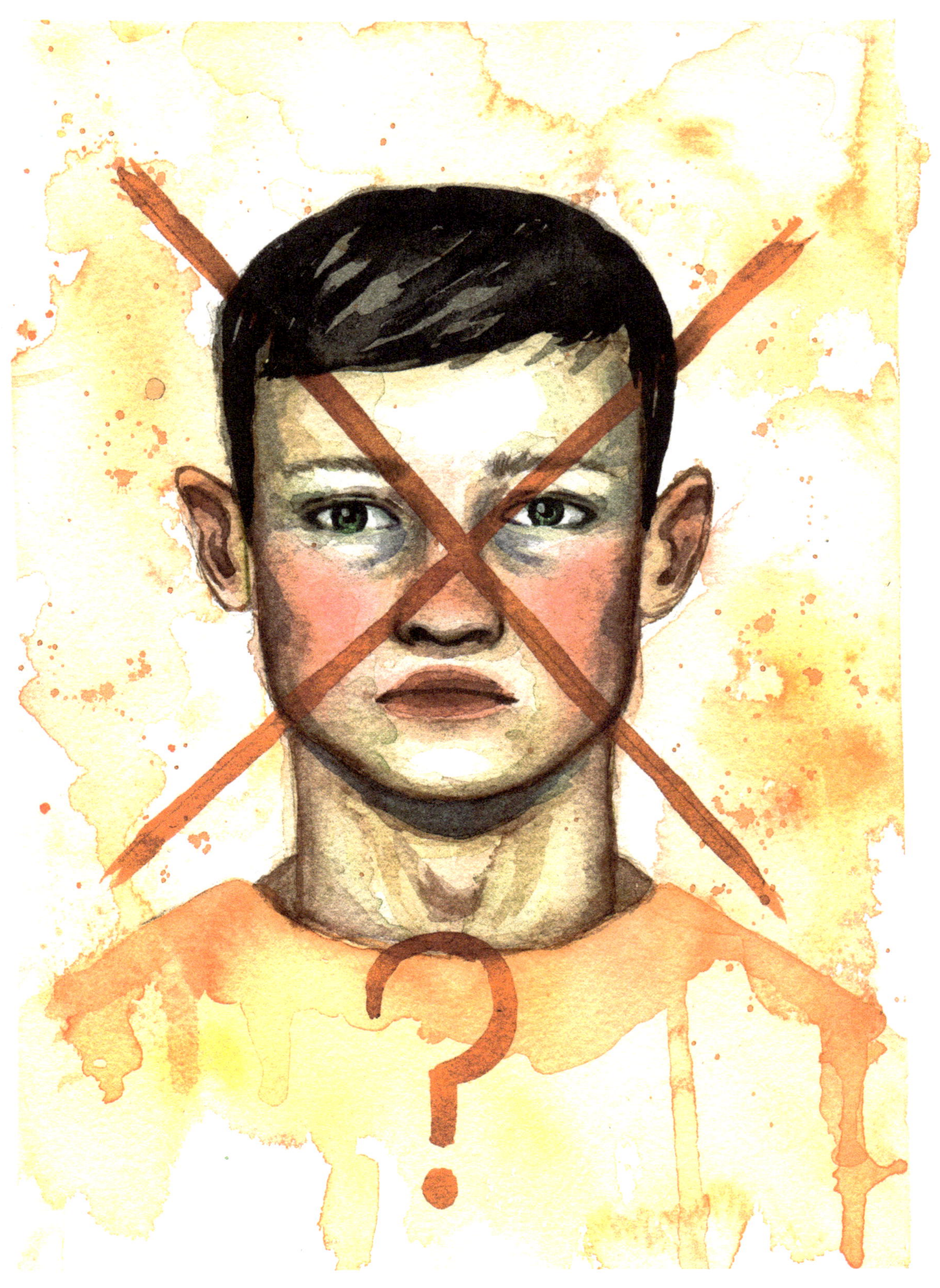

**Breck should not have met someone
he did not know on his own.**

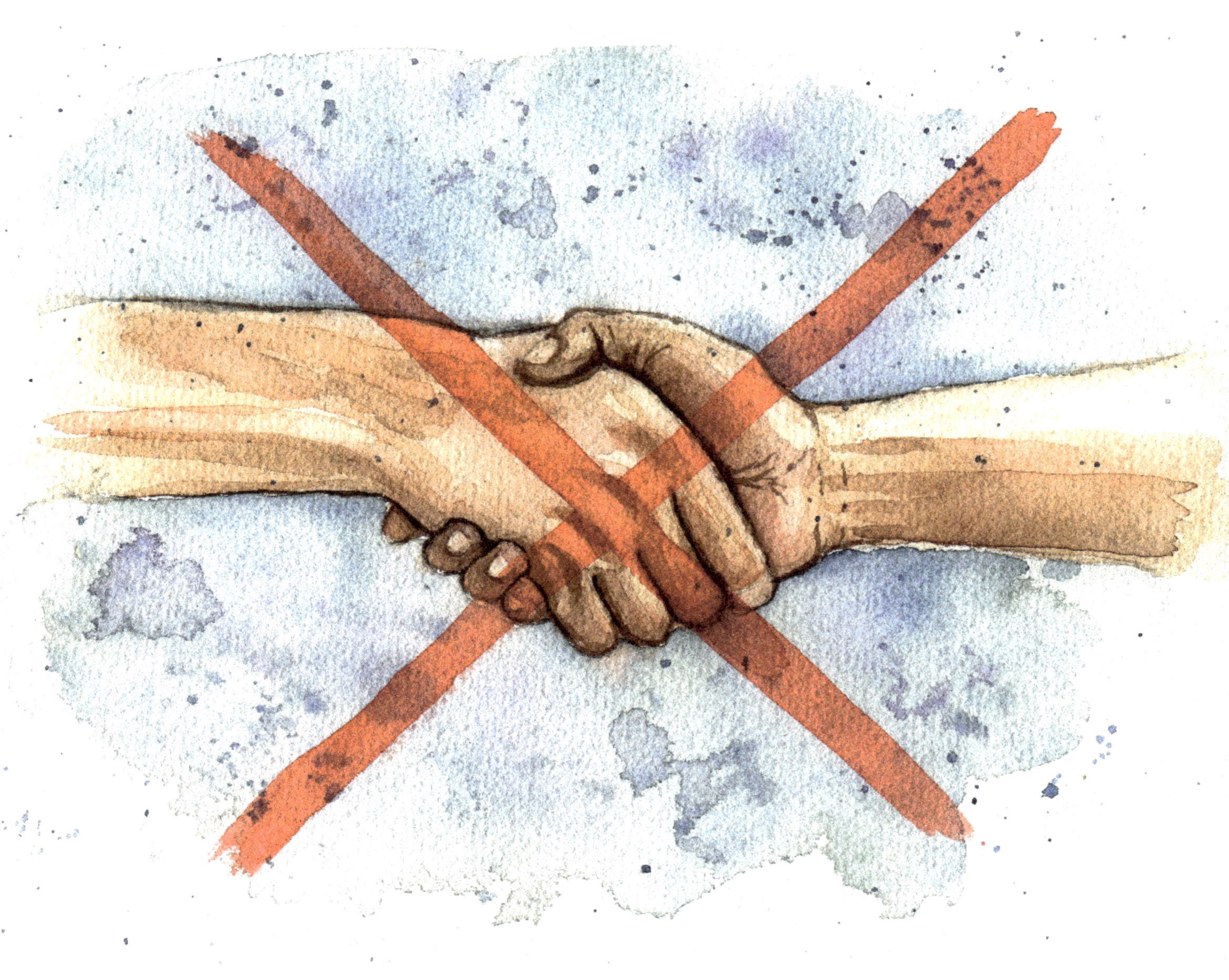

It is okay to let an adult know if you are worried about something or someone on the computer.

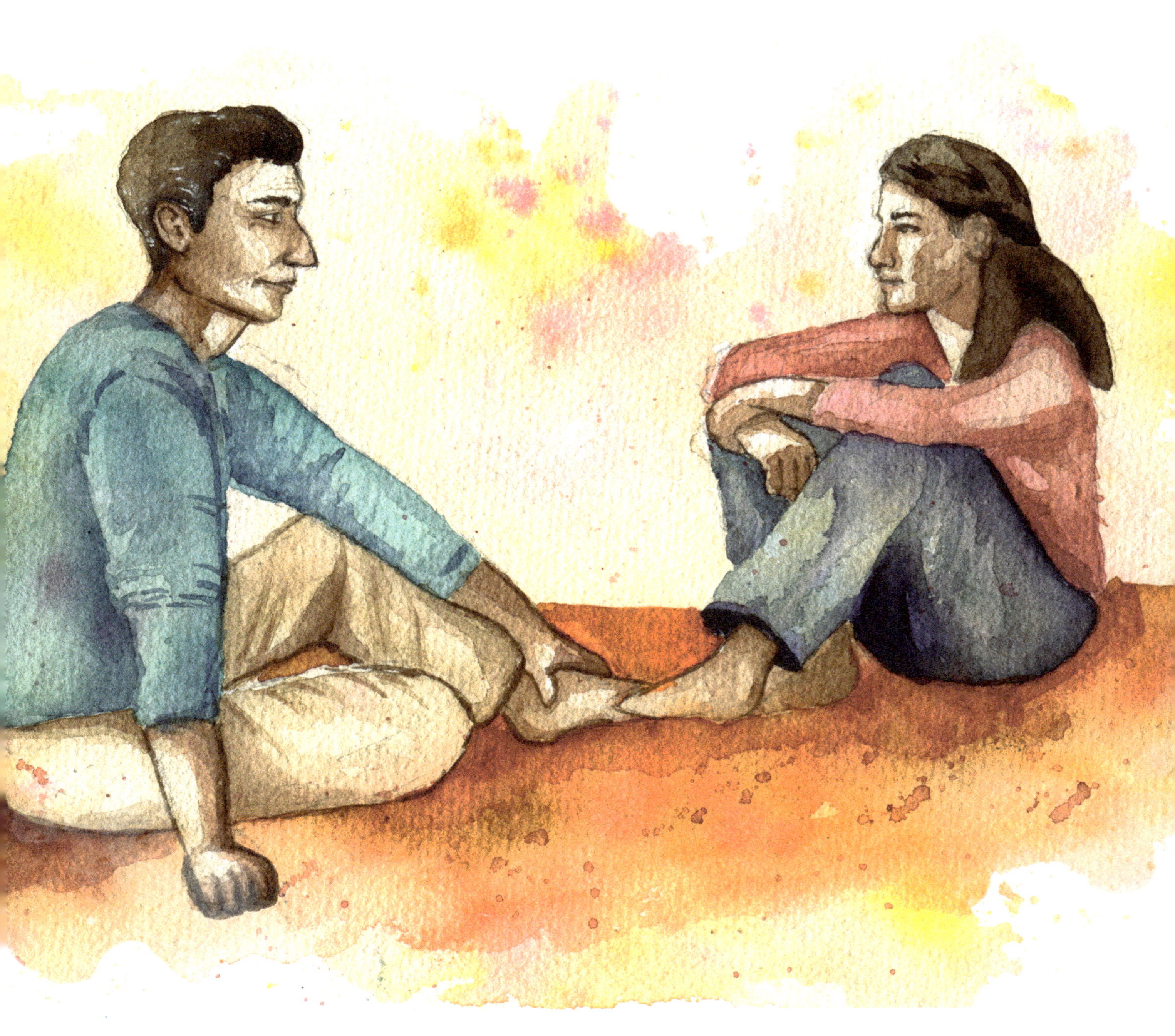

Be safe on the computer and online.

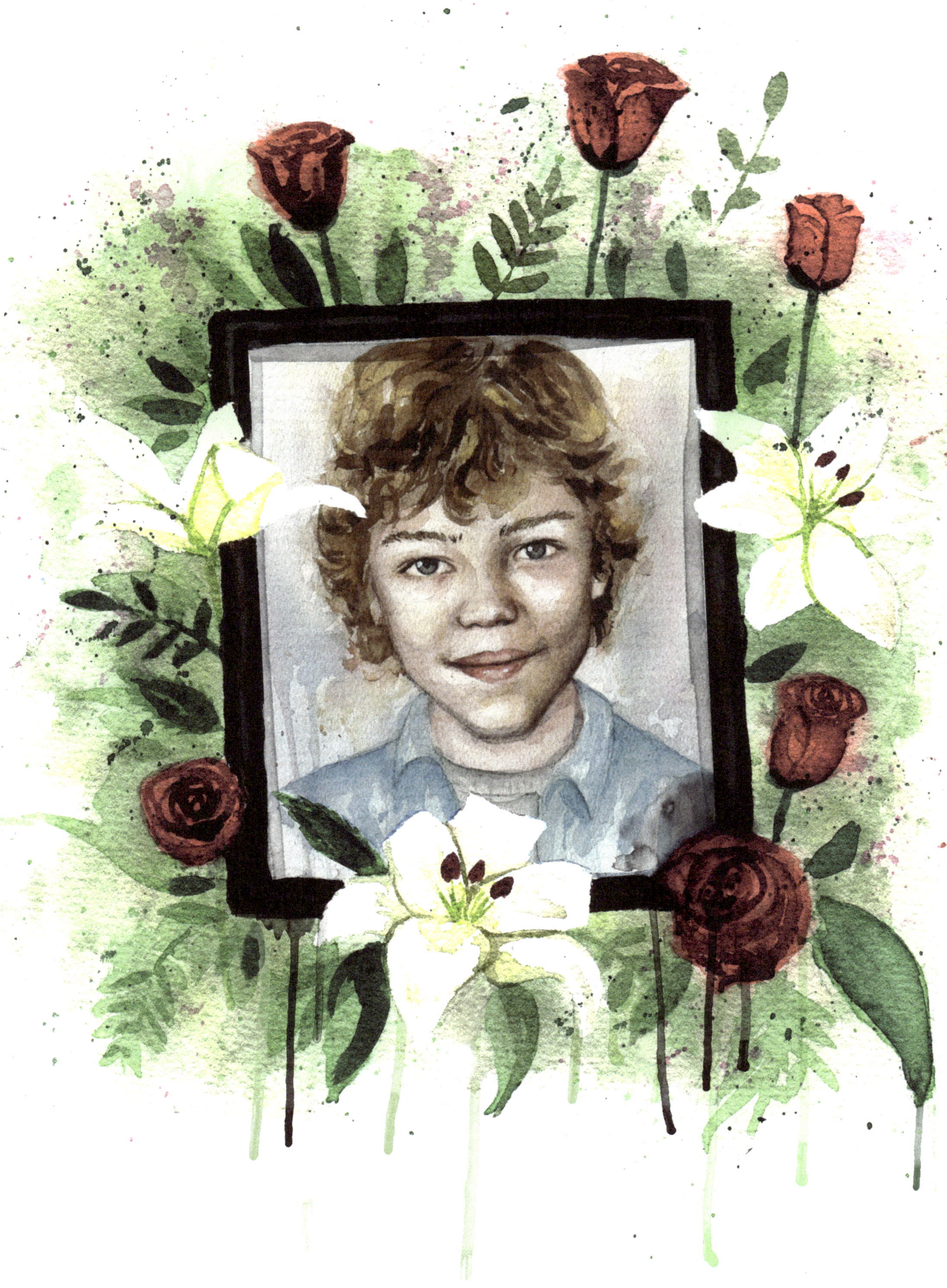

Remember Breck.

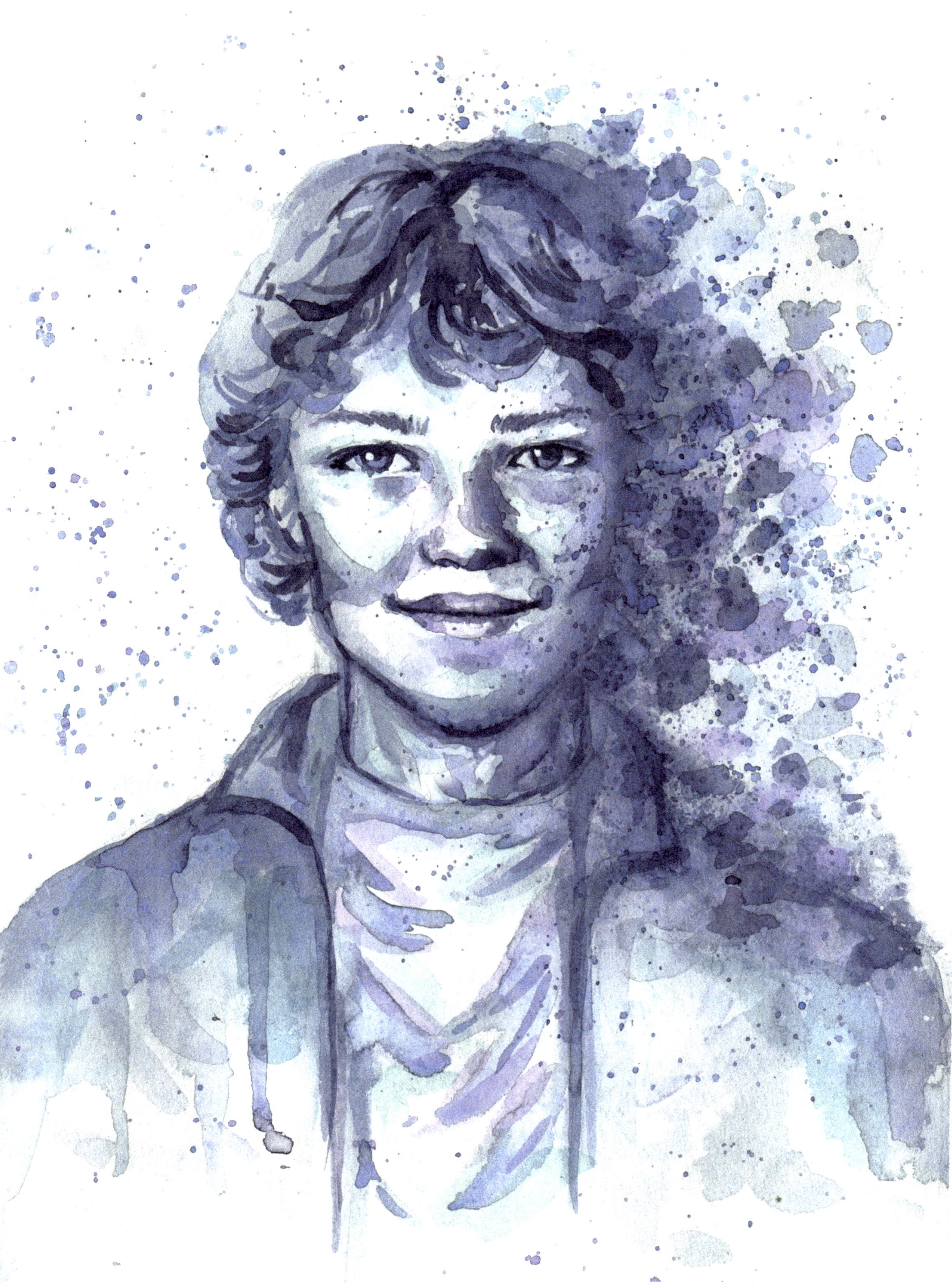

The Breck Principles

The Breck Foundation is raising awareness for playing safe whilst using the internet. Keep safe by following these simple principles that we have created using Breck's name.

Be aware & believe
Be aware of the real dangers we may face online. Believe that there are some people who use the internet with bad intentions.

Report it
Report any concerns immediately to a trusted adult at home or school, Childline, NSPCC, CEOP or police.

Educate & Empower
Educate others on the signs of grooming and exploitation. Be empowered to act on concerns.

Communicate
Communicate with your friends to encourage them to talk about online concerns and ensure everyone looks out for one another.

Know the signs & Keep safe
Know the signs of grooming and exploitation. Keeping safe online must be every-one's priority!

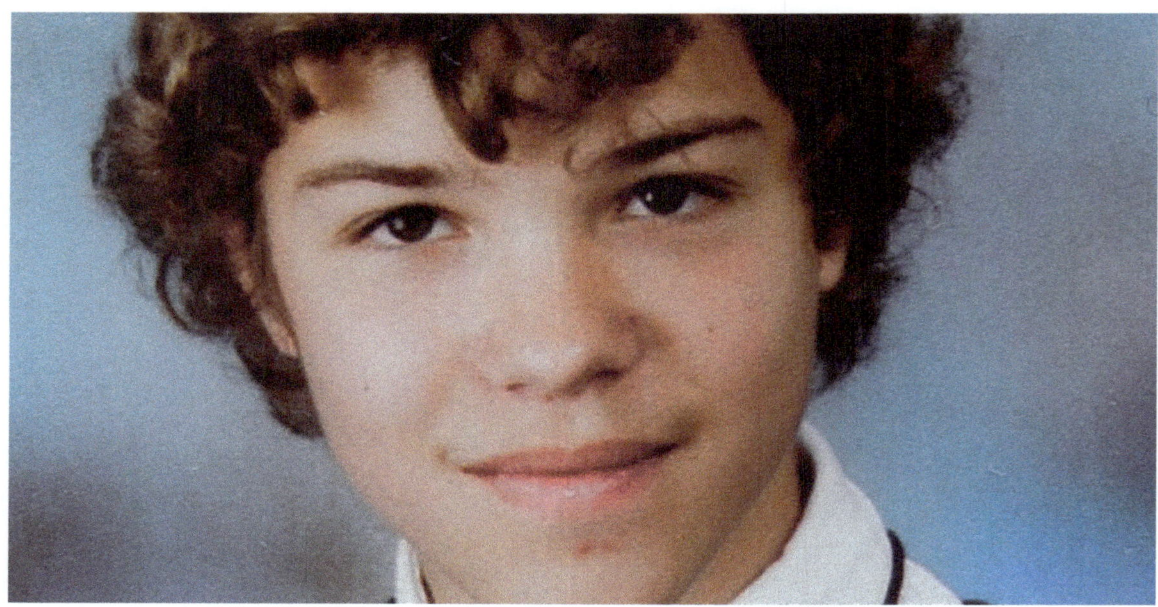

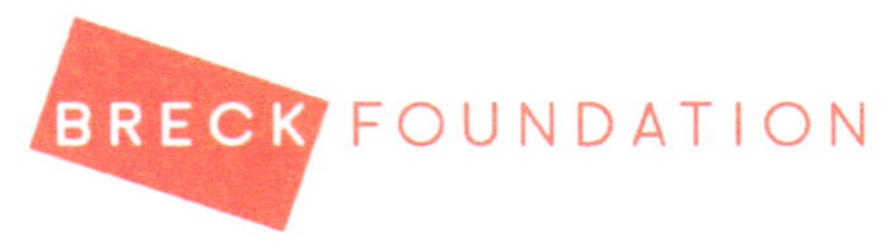

This is Breck Scheme of Work

SUBJECT: PHSE/English/Drama/ICT/Assembly Presentation

TOPIC/UNIT: 'This is Breck': Online Grooming and Keeping Safe

NO. OF LESSONS: 6 Lessons   **Time** 45mins -1 hour

About the Unit:

'This is Breck' is aimed at learners with the cognitive age of 4-8 years old.

The aim of this scheme of work is to introduce the story of the tragedy of Breck Bednar and begin instilling basic online safety and issues around online grooming.

Students will study

- The Story of Breck Bednar
- Good and Bad things about the internet
- What makes a good friend
- Who to talk to talk about worries online
- Feelings involved in grooming
- Presenting and sharing the message of the Breck Foundation

Resources are aimed to be used to support and consolidate learning. Please change writing wherever possible to size, symbol, design to support your students.

The book can be used as a tool to prepare for an assembly or share with another class the information on internet safety. As you go through the story, give students, roles and lines within the text. Equally, you can develop lines and characters to go with what you are presenting.

If a student during the process of studying this text, asks to speak to staff or divulges any issue with safeguarding issues, please follow your facilities safeguarding procedures.

The Breck Foundation is continually developing resources. We are currently developing music/songs that will be available to support students with emotional literacy, and communication of the story. These pieces could be used during or at the end of your story telling or presentations. They could be sung and signed by the groups.

Any work you create or promote on the cause of the Breck Foundation please share with us on social media using @breckfoundation.

For further information and resources please go to **www.breckfoundation.org**

Warning to educators:

Students will be introduced to a simple outline of the events surrounding the death of Breck Bednar.

Please inform parents and guardians that their child will be studying online safety with a focus on the Breck Bednar story. This is due to the wide videos and interviews that are available online and social media. If you feel appropriate, you may want to have a meeting with parents to discuss how parents can support through the learning of this scheme of work. Please see Appendix 1 as a guide to letter to parents and guardians.

Learning Intentions	Teaching Activities	Differentiation/Points to Note	Resources
To understand the story of 'This is Breck' To understand that Breck was a real person	• Introduce that you are going to be studying the book 'This is Breck'. • Ask if anyone knows anything about Breck? • Study the cover of the book - what could the story be about? • Read 'This is Breck'. • Give time for the story to sink in, offer some time for reflection. You could put a piece of music on. • Read the story again and ask the group whether they think that this is a true story or not. • Use Appendix 2: Picture of Breck to show the real Breck. • Explain that this is a true story and this really did happen. • Explain that we are learning this story to keep safe and others safe on the internet. • Use the worksheet Appendix 3. 'This is Breck' Story Match. Students can draw lines to match the statement in the story to the image that matches. • Once students have finished go through the answers to see if learning has been consolidated • At the end of the session, reassure students that the internet is a good thing and this rarely happens but we want to keep them safe. • Ask each student if they are okay or want to share anything about what they have learnt before they leave.	• Please adapt the writing in the books to the size or symbol that is suitable to your class group • Some students may need to stop the lesson and have some further time to process. Please give this extra time and space • Choose wording of computer/internet carefully. Students may think that groomers only work through the internet if you use the phrase internet. Try using computer and internet together. • When using appendix 3. Students can draw lines from the picture to the statement or if developing, motor skills students could cut out the images and statements. These could then be put on a different sheet of paper. Equally, if developing handwriting you could give the images and get the students to write down what they think is going on with the story form the image.	• This is Breck Student or Teacher edition • Appendix 2: Picture of Breck Bednar • Appendix 3: 'This is Breck' Story Match

Learning Intentions	Teaching Activities	Differentiation/Points to Note	Resources
To recall the story of Breck To identify people that can be trusted	• Re-introduce the story of 'This is Breck'. • To do this, 'play the fool' and say you have forgotten the words to the story. See if students one at a time can recall what is going on in the images. • Introduce the idea that you want the students to share what they want with another class or school. Ask students to take on the roles of each character and act out as you read the story. • Give student's time to process the story again. A short music track or reflection time. • Explain to students that the end of the story and what happened could have been very different, if more people had spoken out. Breck's friends all knew about Lewis but none of them told their parents they were worried. • Explain to students that there are adults that we can trust and should tell them things if we are worried or scared about something. • See if any students can come up with a list of trusted people. Use some examples of people that students should not speak to, to consolidate learning. I.e. the woman you sit next to on the public bus. • Use Appendix 4 'People that I can speak to when worried' and Appendix 5 'List of People' for students to select who they think they should talk to when they are worried. Students can cut out the names and stick them onto the sheet. • After the worksheet is complete, get students to share who their trusted adults are. • Before dismissal assure students that if they are worried or scared, it is important to share with any of the trusted adults they have chosen.	• Please adapt the writing in the books to the size or symbol that is suitable to your class group • When telling the story you may want to begin using props to tell the story • When introducing the idea of people that the students can trust you may want to use pictures of different people include images of the students' parents or guardians where possible. • When working on the worksheet Appendix 4. Change to symbol's where needed or get students to write out their answers. Students can also use names of people to. Some students may prefer to prefer to use photographs of the people that they trust too.	• This is Breck Student or Teacher edition • Appendix 4: People I can speak to when I am worried. • Appendix 5: List of people • Glue • Scissors • Pen (optional)

Learning Intentions	Teaching Activities	Differentiation/Points to Note	Resources
To recall the story of Breck To recall who the trusted people are To understand the good and bad issues of the internet and computing	• Begin by asking the students who one of their trusted people are. • Remind students that we should share our worries and fears with computing with everyone. • Ask one student to take the lead on teaching the story and see if they can get it right. • Remind students that they are going to share what they have learnt with other students in the school • Select students who are going to play each role. • Re- read the story 'This is Breck'. Ask the students if they would like time out between. • If you feel the students need it give them reflection time, • When you come back together as a group get a large piece of paper. On one side write good and on the other bad. • Ask students to think of what good things computers and the internet are used for. Write any ideas down that are shared. • Afterwards flip the paper round, use it to highlight the bad things the internet and computing can be used for. Get students to think about Breck's story what bad things happened to him. • Students can then use Appendix 5 and 6 to consolidate their learning. Students can cut and stick the words where they feel is appropriate. • At the end of the lesson, reassure students that computers and the internet are great tools. Few people in the world use them to hurt other people. Remind students that if there is something that is upsetting them, they should speak to a trusted adult.	• Please adapt the writing in the books to the size or symbol that is suitable to your class group. • When using Appendix 6, Students can write on the sheet rather than stick.	• This is Breck Student or Teacher edition • Large piece of paper • Board Marker • Appendix 6: Good and Bad things about computing and the internet • Appendix 7: Words for good and bad things about computing and internet. • Glue • Scissors • Pen (optional)

Learning Intentions	Teaching Activities	Differentiation/Points to Note	Resources
To understand the story of Breck To develop presentation skills To understand what a good friend looks like	• Begin with reminding students that you are presenting the story to other students/classes. • Remind students that they are educating others too. • Rehearse your presentation by telling the story and the students acting it out. • You may want to rehearse/practice this 2 or 3 times. • If students need reflection, time after this, offer it to them with music or quiet. • When the group comes together. Ask the question, 'What makes a good friend?' • After the students have had some time to think, act for students a bad friend. i.e. lying to a friend, pressuring them to do stuff, saying horrible things, hurting them. • Make sure that your students all understand that what you have presented is wrong. • Get the students to then work in pairs to show what a good friend looks like. • Get students to share their ideas. • Explain to students that Lewis in the story was not being a good friend. Ask students to identify reasons why Lewis was not a good friend to Breck • Then use Appendix 8: What makes a good friend? And Appendix 9: What makes a good friend? Ideas. Students may want to write their own initial ideas down. Students can cut and stick what ideas they feel make a good friend. • At the end of the lesson get students to share what they think makes a good friend. • Remind students that most people want to be friendly but if you feel your friend is not being nice to you, you must talk to a trusted adult.	• Please adapt the writing in the books to the size or symbol that is suitable to your class group. • You might want to have scenarios ready for students about being a good friend. • When using Appendix 8 and 9 you may want to get students to write ideas themselves.	• This is Breck Student or Teacher edition • Any props you are using to support the story telling • Appendix 8: What makes a good friend? • Appendix 9: What makes a good friend? Ideas • Glue • Scissors • Pen (optional)

Learning Intentions	Teaching Activities	Differentiation/Points to Note	Resources
To create a play from the story 'This is Breck' To develop emotional understanding	• Begin by reminding students you are going to share what they have learnt with someone, a class, the school in the next week. • Pretend that you have forgotten what happens in your students' play. Ask students to present the play to you. • Give students feedback on how you think their play went. • Get students to rehearse again with your feedback. • If needed give children time to reflect, this can be to music. • When you come back in a group, ask them to make a general list of as many feelings as they can. • Ask students how they feel right now and get them to feedback. • Get the students to split into three groups. Give each group a person: Lorin (Brecks Mum), Lewis and Breck. • Rotate every 3 minutes asking the students how this person may feel about what happened to them during the story. • Share the separate group's ideas with the whole class. • Students can then individually use Appendix 10: How might they feel and Appendix 11: Feelings. Students can cut out and stick the different feeling that that they may have during the story. • Ask students to leave the one about themselves to last. • With the last one, ask students to write down how they feel when they hear the story about Breck. • At the end of the lesson, discuss with the students that it is good to talk about our feelings and that is good to share how we feel. Remind students if they have worries or fears they should discuss with a trusted adult.	• Please adapt the writing in the books to the size or symbol that is suitable to your class group • When working in groups as to how each might feel, it might be better for your class to work as a whole rather than separate groups. • Students may want to write their own answers on the work sheet.	• This is Breck Student or Teacher edition • Any props you are using to support the story telling • Large piece of paper • Appendix 10: How might they feel and Appendix 11: Feelings • Board marker • Glue • Scissors • Pen (optional)

Learning Intentions	Teaching Activities	Differentiation/Points to Note	Resources
To teach others the story of Breck To consolidate learning To share the Breck Foundation message	• At this point students should have presented their work to someone, a class or school. • Firstly, congratulate students on doing a good job. • Share with students, videos or images from their presentation. • Using Appendix 12: Storyboard - Use photos of the student's presentation and get students to re-write the story of what happened to Breck. • Once work is complete, discuss with students that you are going to send their work to the Breck Foundation @ breckfoundation (on social media) to show what they have taught others about the Breck story. • After this, evaluate with students all they have learnt over the previous weeks. • Good and Bad computing and internet, • Trusted people and why we have them • Feeling that may come when things go wrong • Finally remind the students that what happened to Breck is extremely rare, however we are trying to keep as many people safe as possible. Remind them that this was a real story and that if any of the students have any worries, they must talk to a trusted adult.	• Please adapt the writing in the books to the size or symbol that is suitable to your class group • Appendix 12 can also be drawn by the students • If Appendix 12 is not suitable, you may want to create a poster for the Breck foundation, a photo montage of the students' work.	• Permission for students images to be used on social media • Appendix 12 • Camera • Images or Video of the students presenting • Glue • Scissors

Identified Opportunities for ICT: Any or all parts of this scheme of work can be transferred to computer.
Please feel free to adapt and change to fit the needs of your students.

Helping the Breck Foundation: Please share with us any work, presentations, assemblies, work that students create and displays. Please make sure that you have all necessary permissions before sending anything to us. Please share with us on our social media @breckfoundation or please email one of the team. We are developing our resources continually and like to see what ideas you come up with when sharing the story. Please look on our website for further resources and information, including videos, music and ways to support the foundation further. www.breckfoundation.org

Appendix 1

Letter to Parents and Guardians regarding intoduction to 'This is Breck'

Dear Parent or Guardian

Over the next 6 weeks your child will studying online safety and online grooming. Therefore we will be using the book 'This is Breck' as our focus.

This book is aimed to introduce students to online grooming and issues around internet safety. It is based on the true story of Breck Bednar. Breck was a 14 year old boy who was groomed and murdered by a 17 year old who Breck thought was his friend.

Your child over the next coming weeks may have further questions and may want to discuss what happened to Breck. There are lots of interviews and information online and on social meida about Breck and you may want to filter what is seen and read by your child.

We recommend that the book 'This is Breck' is a good place to start with discussing this topic. A storybook edition is available to order online and and you can find out more information about Breck and the work of the charity the Breck Foundation on http://www.breckfoundation.org/

I will be arranging a meeting with parents and guardians on ________________________ to discuss and go through the scheme of work. Please let me know if you are able to attend or have any further questions about this scheme of work.

We thank you for your continued support

Regards

Appendix 2

Picture of the real Breck Bednar in Year 9

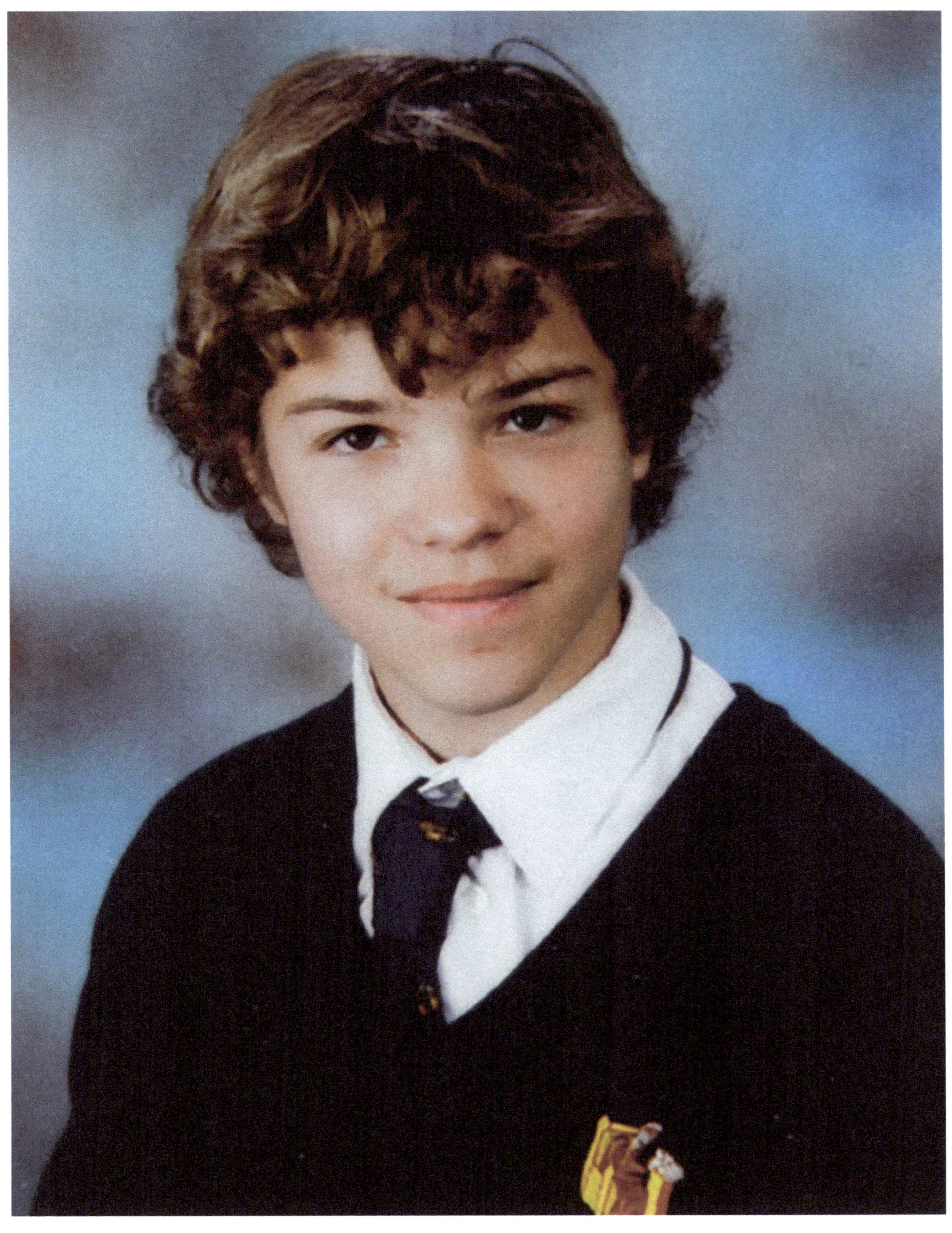

Appendix 3:

'This is Breck' Story Match

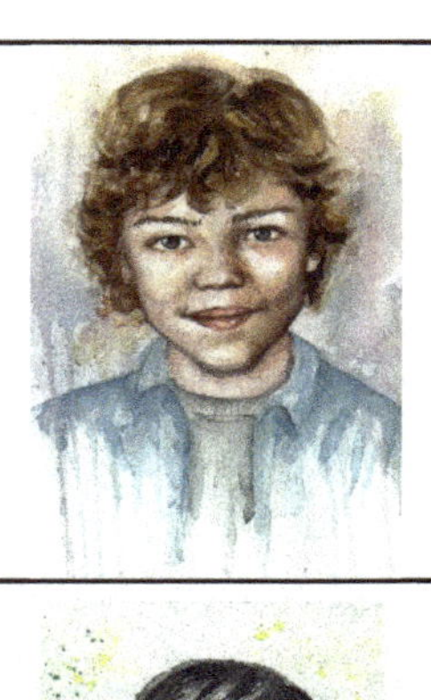

Breck's Mum didn't like Lewis. Breck and his Mum argued.

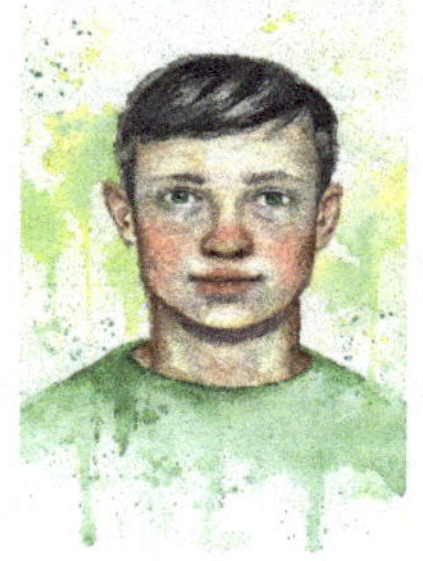

Breck made a friend on the computer called Lewis. Lewis lied about who he was.

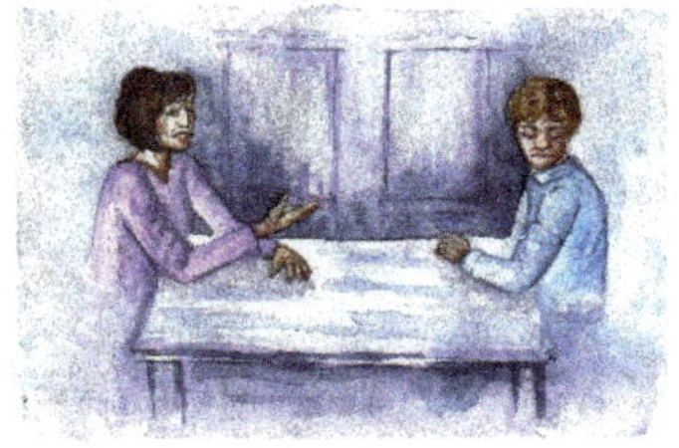

It is important to keep safe online and talk to a trusted adult if you are worried about something you have seen online

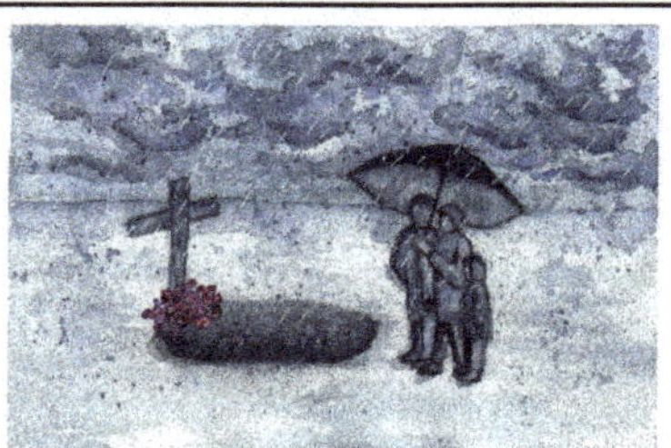

Lewis killed Breck. Breck's Family are very sad.

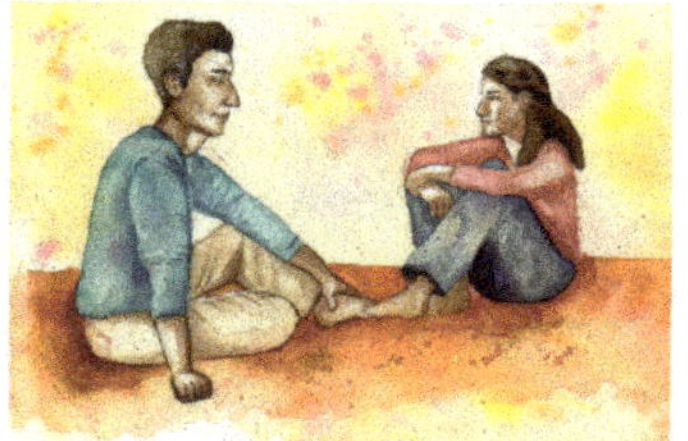

Breck was a young boy who liked playing on the computer.

Appendix 4

People I can talk to if I am worried.

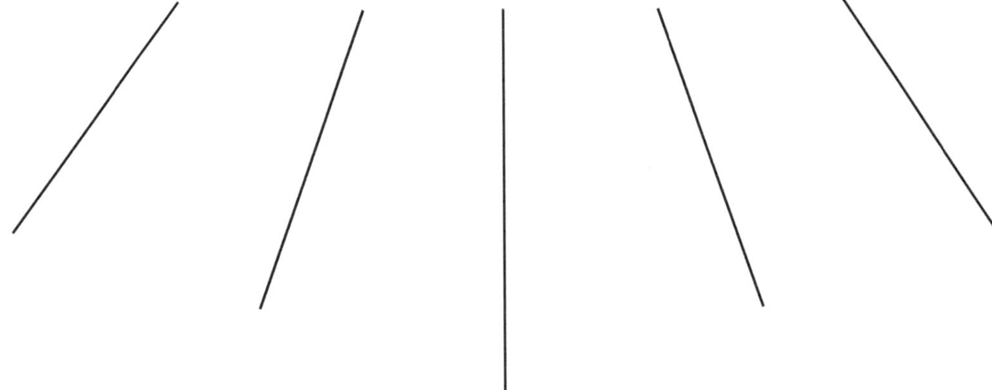

Appendix 5

List of people

Mum	Dad	Brother
Sister	Grandparents	Doctor
Teacher	Teaching Assistant	Police Officer
Social Worker	Carer	Auntie/Uncle
Shop Assistant	The lady next door to you on the bus	Your friend

Appendix 6

Good and Bad things about Computing, Gaming and Internet

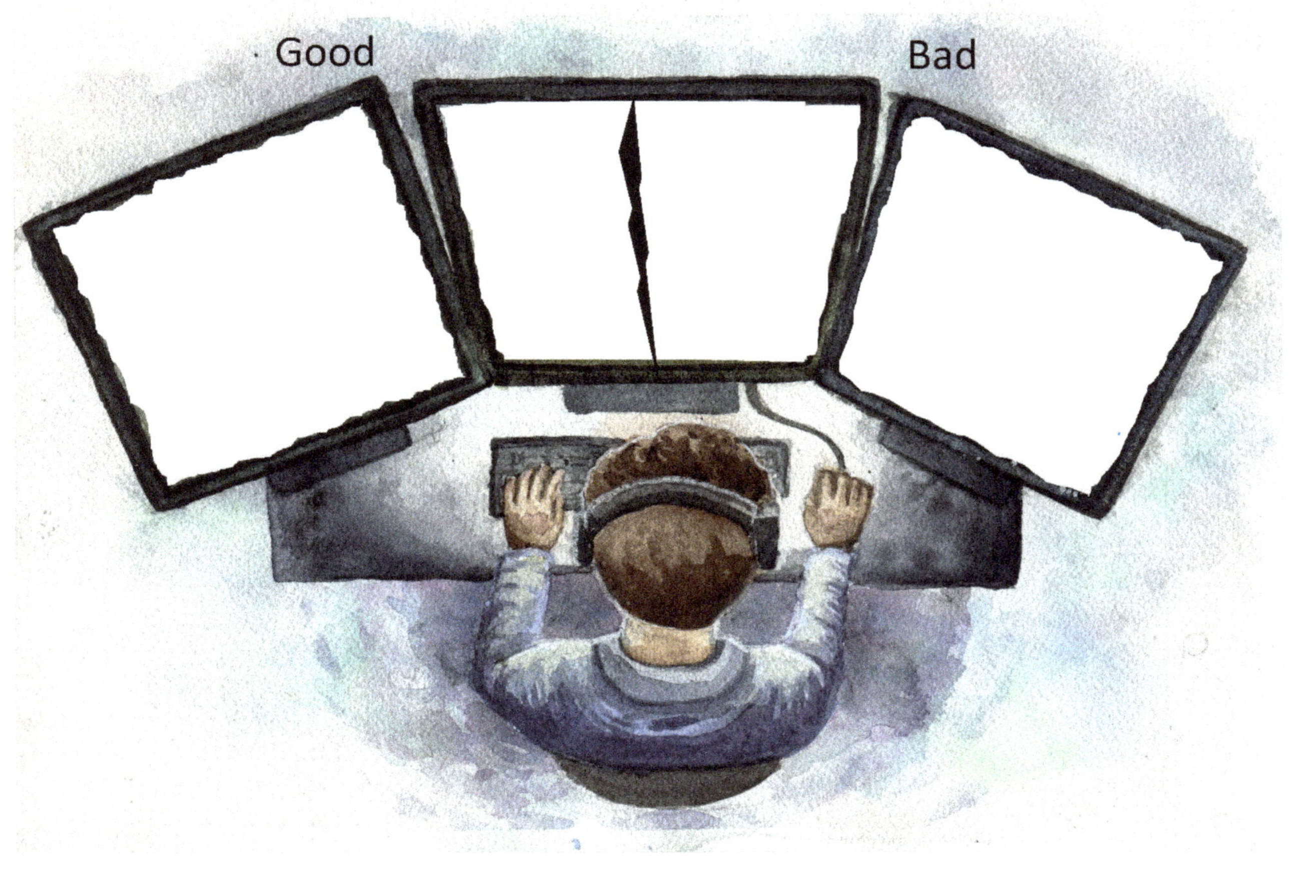

Appendix 7

Words for Good and Bad computing and internet

Gaming with people you don't know	Doing work	Keeping in contact with friends and family
Speaking to people you don't know	Arranging to meet with people you don't know	Sending pictures to someone you don't know
Doing homework	Watching videos	Listening to music
Finding out information	Videos that are inapproriate	Spending lots of time online

Appendix 8

What makes a good friend?

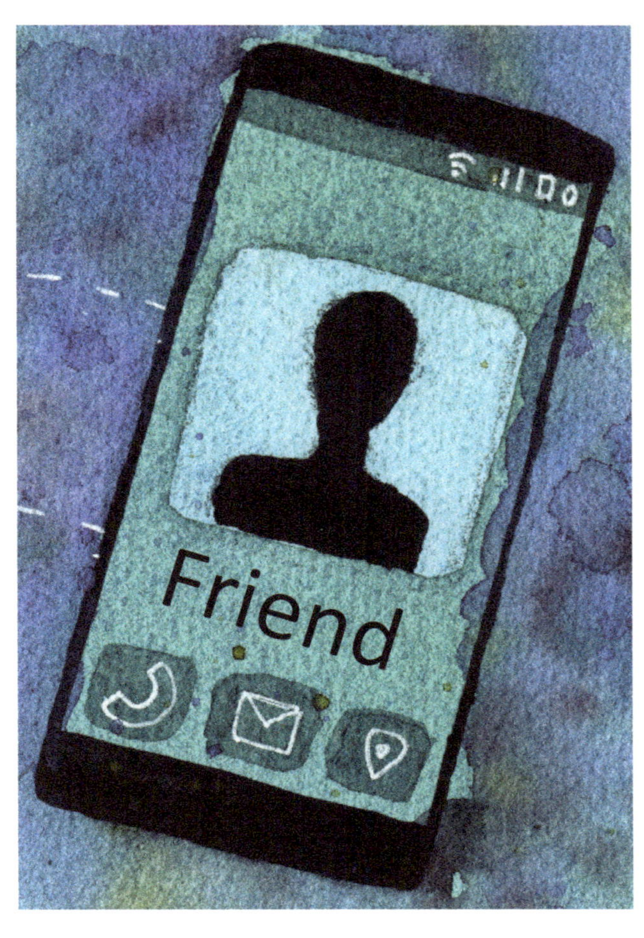

Appendix 9

What makes a good friend? Ideas

Have the same interests	Someone who you have met	Someone whose picture you have seen
Someone who doesn't tell you to do bad things	Likes talking to you in person	You have known for a long time
Someone who is nice to your other friends and family	Tells you not to like your family	Makes you feel sad
Makes you feel happy	Makes you change who you are	Likes you as you are

Appendix 10

How might they feel?

<table>
<tr><td>Brecks Mum (Lorin)</td><td>Lewis</td></tr>
<tr><td>Breck</td><td>You
(stick a picture of yourself here)</td></tr>
</table>

Appendix 11

Feelings

Sad	Angry	Confused
Lost	Happy	Lonely
Controlling	Mean	Excited
Trusting	Awful	Worried
Powerful	Scared	Strong

Appendix 12

Storyboard

www.ingramcontent.com/pod-product-compliance
Ingram Content Group UK Ltd.
Pitfield, Milton Keynes, MK11 3LW, UK
UKHW062115150726
7214IPUK00025B/420